Two Shamans and a Healer

Healing the Heart of a Nation

And an Introduction to Holographic Programming,
Programming of the Universal Hologram is Now Possible.

Paul Barbaro – Health Researcher

Hands-On-Healing Pioneer

First Edition

ISBN - 13: 978-1495373602

ISBN - 10: 1495373606

BISAC: Health & Fitness / Healing / Programming / Holograms

Two Shamans and a Healer

Healing the Heart of a Nation

Published by:
Healing Hedgehog Press
20044 Pacifica Drive,
Cupertino, CA 95014

Email us today at healingangelguides@yahoo.com
We'd love to hear from you.

Web Site with TV shows, trainings;
and testimonials - www.healingangelguides.com

(408) 253-6577 Office Phone, please leave a message
if we are out.

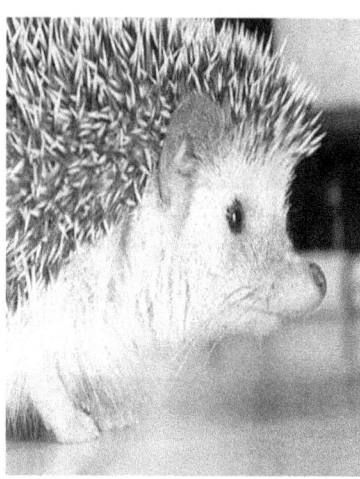

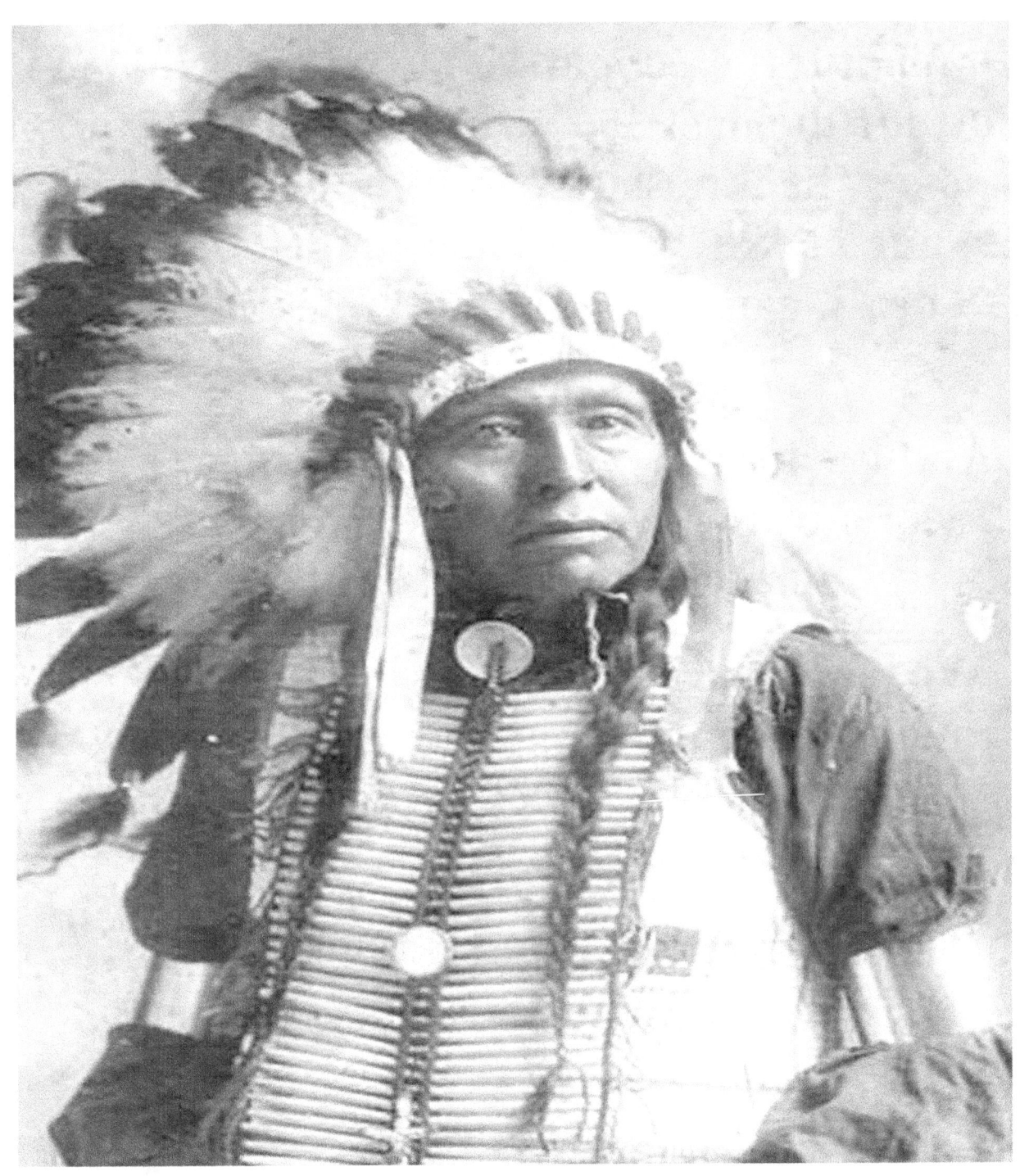

Honoring of Ancestor, Chief Seattle, photo c1850

What if the people we have been killing off for the past 300 years hold the solution to our health issues, and to the healing of our bodies, of healing our societies, of healing our Nation and of healing the Earth?

And isn't it time we cherished the wisdom of our own Native People instead of persecuting our differences?

We teach that the healing of our nation is connected to the languages and customs of our Native Peoples, whom are our national treasures, and;

There are still a few of them left that we can listen to, and learn their wisdom. There is time, it's not too late, and there is still hope…

Who or What is a Shaman?

Within many societies a shaman refers to a spiritual doctor or priest who restores balance and wholeness to the soul. The Shaman is able to bring guidance and mend illnesses of the human soul caused by traumatic experiences in current or past lives. Shamans occupy a position between the seen and the unseen (spiritual) worlds. They are healers. Even when they look or sound different, or have a spiritual connection with the Earth, a wise person might connect with them and learn their ways. Could it possibly help?

Healing Your Soul with a Shaman

In the United States a growing population is learning the benefits of healing the soul to bring increased health, happiness, and even prosperity to their current life. Those devoted to spiritual lives, such as Buddhists Monks, and Native American Shamans appreciate that restoring the soul will benefit future lifetimes. This is a very enlightened spiritual understanding and path.

The soul retains all experiences. The process of restoring the soul is similar to peeling off layers of an onion. This requires the use of a combination of healings. The intention is to remove emotional impact and patterns caused by painful events. The Shaman operates primarily within the spiritual world, which in turn affects the human world. Some Americans chose to study the culture and wisdom we lost when the Native Americans world was destroyed. Is it possible that they had wisdom that would help us in today's world?

This Healing Process Came from Native American Wisdom

Thank God that I had the encounters with these Native Americans when I was needing this information the most. This entire healing method of inviting your ancestors, angels, guides, saints, family and friends, plus inviting their "tribes" to join the healing adds power to the process.

Two Shamans & A Healer
Healing the Heart of a Nation

I, this author, was an energy healer since 1982, and I thought I was "pretty good." Except that the people closest to me were dying, my brother Mark, and my sister Mary, my Uncle Victor and later my Uncle Joe, my best friends Randy H., David S., Cam S., Yvonne G., Fred H., and eight more very close friends. These people were good beings and I feel they had twenty to forty good years left in them when they died so young. I realized that I did not have all the answers, and I needed to find what I was lacking in my knowledge and in my healing method. I believed that true healing existed on earth and I was out to find it.

I had been asking Western and Asian healers for thirty years "What are the keys to healing the body?" Their answers were often complex and unsatisfying. A good friend and mentor of mine, Dr. George Carr, M.D., gave me the wonderful advice to continue asking until I get satisfying answers to my questions. He taught me that, "There is only one Truth, and all information aligns with the top of the <u>Truth Pyramid</u>." He taught me to "Always seek the Truth." Few pieces of advice have served me as well as these have.

My First Shaman & Teacher Encounter

On a bright but chilly summer day outside of Anchorage, Alaska, in July of 2008, I was watching hang-gliders gently float on summer thermals having launched from a tall peak. It was a lazy, relaxing day. As I watched large birds and hang-gliders floating I noticed a Native American doing what appeared to be a ceremony in the center of a large Alaskan meadow. I am an inquisitive healer, and I knew an opportunity when I saw one. When the Native American was done with his ritual, I approached him and introduced myself. He told me that his name is Running Deer. After pleasantries I asked him about Native American healing methods. I was not prepared for what he told me.

I asked Running Deer, "Among all the chakras, pressure points and meridians on the body, which are the most important?" He told me, "There are six spots on the body that release the energy of past trauma much faster than all the others." He pointed to these areas on his body saying, "They are the forehead, the chest (front) heart, and the don-tien on the front of the body, and the occipitals, the back heart, and the sacrum on the back of the body. These are the 'Hottest spots on the body, and healers get the best results eliminating early trauma by focusing on these spots."

So I asked him, "How is this early trauma released through these six spots?"

He replied, "Your hands are like jumper cables. Touching these locations lets the energy drain out [brings balance]. He then said, "All healing is balance and grounding.""

I asked him if that is why he was barefoot when he was doing his ceremony, and he said, "Yes." I felt that this was good information but I had no idea how to implement it into my healing practice.

The Wise Shaman Said, "All Healing is Balance and Grounding."

Important Note: *You are **not** putting energy into your partner. You are just discharging old stuck energy from their past. There is a big difference. When energy is put into ones body, and there is stuck energy that has not been balanced, it just further "balls up the stuck energy." It is not good to add energy to stuck energy. I avoid people who want to "put energy" into me or anyone else. A word to the wise.*

The Second Important Shaman & Teacher

More healing enlightenment came from a Muscogee-Creek Shaman named Charles Hawkins, a.k.a. "Crowman," from Santa Cruz, California. His credentials are that when he was a youth he was in a high speed auto accident. He was in the hospital for a full year recuperating. In his states of unconsciousness he made his connection with Universal mind. A shaman goes between the seen and unseen worlds. They are teachers and spiritual guides. They carry forward the traditions of their tribes.

Crowman and I had been friends for several years and one day after a healing session, I asked Crowman, "When the medicine man is in the teepee with a Native person who is sick or injured, and stretched out on the cot, with a small fire in the center and the smoke is going, and the medicine man is doing his dance with a rattle or drum, and he is chanting 'Hi-Yaa, Hi-Yaa, Hi-Yaa!' for hours on end, what's really going on?"

Crowman told me, "He's calling on the person's ancestors, guides, masters, angels, and family members, basically the injured person's tribe. And I call on my own tribe, to be included into the healing session/energy because we are all connected."

Inquisitively I asked, "Isn't that a terrible waste of a medicine man's precious time, he has so many other patients to work on (and he only has seven minutes to spend with each one, considering the present model of medicine)?"

I thought I was being smart with my question. The wise shaman became very quiet and said in a soft voice, "We heal as a tribe or group. If your tribe is sick, you will not remain well." Then he said, "You need to include your ancestors, guides, masters, family and angels in your healing because they might not have had the spiritual healing techniques that we have today. Besides your ancestors and your spiritual family have a vested interest in your well-being because part of their job is to cover your back, keep you safe, and watch out for your survival. They survive through you, like it or not." This was totally new information to me.

Then I said to Crowman, "I don't know a lot of my ancestors, and I really don't care for some of my family and relatives."

He said, "That doesn't matter. Just include them anyway, don't compromise your healing by excluding anyone."

Then I had the bright idea to asked him, "Do all the indigenous people of earth know this wisdom?"

Crowman said, "Yes."

I then asked, "Why have the indigenous people of earth not given the 'pale faces' this information before now?"

The 68 year old Crowman said, "No one ever asked before now." And then he added, "The 'pale faces' were too busy killing us off to ask what we knew. Indigenous people have a tremendous wealth of knowledge about the earth, life, harmony, energy, balance and healing."

The wise shaman said, "We heal as
a tribe or group. If your tribe is sick,
you will not remain well." And,
"You need to include your ancestors, guides,
masters, family and angels in your healing because
they might not have had the spiritual healing
techniques that we have today. Your ancestors and
your spiritual
family have a vested interest in your
well being and survival.
They survive through you,
like it or not."

What a shock! There was nothing within me that was prepared for this profound wisdom. In an instant my whole understanding of healing shifted upward into a whole new realm. Do you see the information you can get by simply and persistently asking questions until you get a satisfying answer? When these two pieces of information "hit me" and I "got it" my entire world shifted, and I was in a different range of effectiveness as a healer.

This healing system came directly from this information provided by heaven through the mouths of these wise older shamans. I thank God for the wisdom of the indigenous native peoples. Left to ourselves I doubt if we ever would have found this system.

I firmly believe that with this healing method recovery time can be significantly reduced, and hospitals can save on cost of care. It's a, "Win for the hospitals – and a win for the patients!"

A Story of Forgiveness

Note: *I was so focused on his healing wisdom that I missed the importance of this next piece of my conversation with Crowman.*

Then I asked Crowman, "Can you forgive the 'pale faces' for their ignorance, and their crimes against your Nations for these many years?"

Crowman thought for a minute and said, "Yes."

We need to remember that the Native Americans think globally. It isn't just one "Native American" – it's "All Native Americans, all tribes, all indigenous peoples, together." The white man, and all people everywhere are part of this global thinking. There is no separation. This is inclusive thinking.

So in order to be inquisitively inclusive I asked Crowman, "All White Men, All Native Americans, all indigenous peoples all over the world, for all time, and all crimes and injustices committed by those White Men and those indigenous people's crimes against the Whites, and against each other?

Crowman, who had the authority to speak for those groups thought for a moment, and he said, "Yes."

Then I asked Crowman, "So is it okay to move forward from our past history of injury, injustice and crimes on each other?"

Crowman said, "Yes."

> **The importance of his answer is that I firmly believe that, at that moment, Crowman forgave all White Men for all their trespasses against all tribes, all Native Americans, all indigenous peoples all over the world for all the injustices and crimes of the past for all time.**

It is important to let people know that it is okay to move forward from our past (European) history.

Note: These front pages are laid out for effective display on Amazon's web site. These are the core messages of this book presented here. My hope is to spark interest in healing chronic pain, especially persistent psycho-somatic pain rooted in early childhood trauma.

People ask me, "Why would you write another book on healing? Aren't their enough books already?"

No! In a bookstore with ten-thousand different books on healing, this is the only one that deals with Universal Holographic Programming. This healing method makes your body's energy system and healing easy to understand, easy to do, and where one can study it in one day, do the method as it is taught, and see a result that same day.* That has not existed before this book and this method. In this world where everything seems to be instant. This method is as close to instant as one can get. You are worth the results. You are worth being healthy. Your loved ones are worth the results and the increased health. The processes in this book are worth your serious consideration, time and effort.

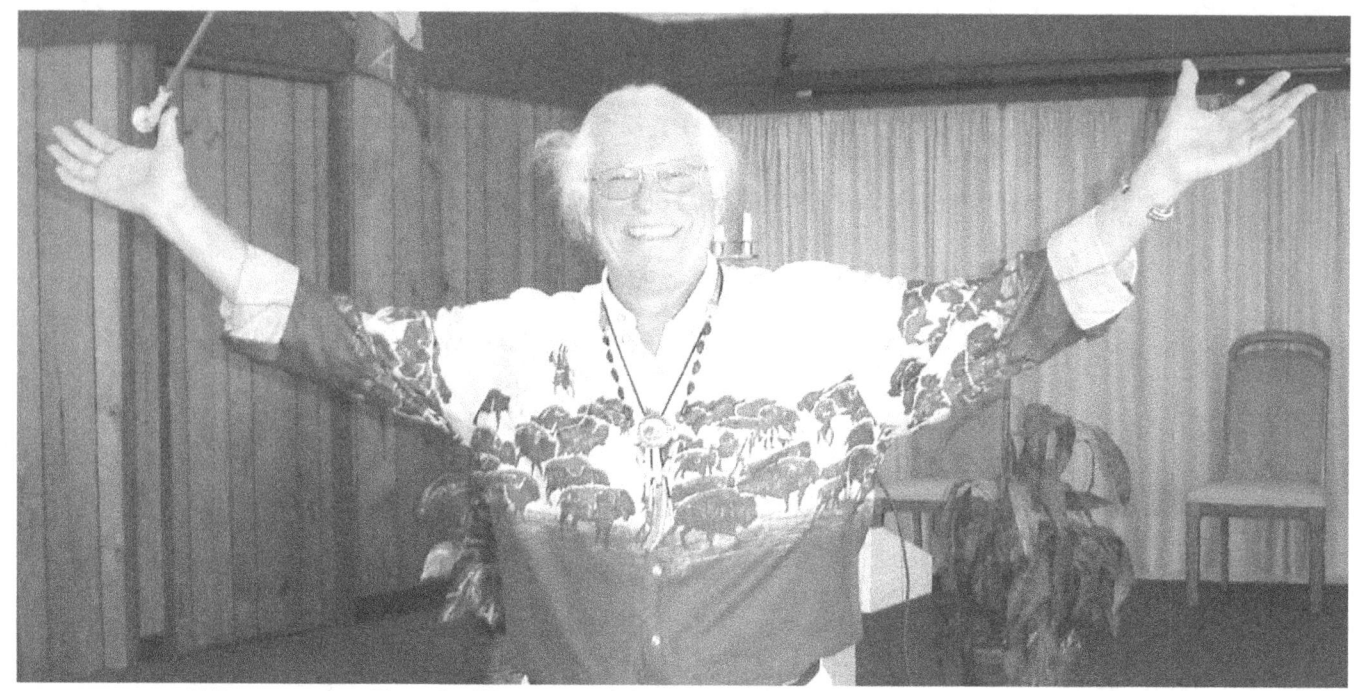

Muscogee-Creek Shaman, Crowman, a.k.a. Charles Hawkins

Tribal Healing and It's Importance for You

There is a reciprocal effect for taking responsibility for healing one's tribe. Tribal and ancestral trauma is expressed in your DNA. DNA can be seen as the ultimate cellular memory. That memory is so complete that it created you. This healing system uses and relies upon your angels, ancestors, masters, guides, and present family for your healing because we heal as a tribe. You do not have to believe this because this system works independent of personal belief. Once the early trauma is discharged, balanced, neutralized, and thus eliminated, there is no foundation, engine, nor energy to power later pain. This healing system balances that early pain energy and makes healing much easier. Healing equals balance. Balance equals flowing energy in the body. Balance and healing is good. Stuck energy promotes illness. Taking responsibility for your health and energy is good. This balance heals the past and the future generations. This is important to know. Balance is in the present. Healing is in the present. Taking responsibility for your tribe's healing gives you a special blessing of long lasting healing for you and your children and tribe. Your ancestor's energy is healed because you invited them into your healing session and asked them to resolve their past health issues. Asking ancestors and providing a pathway for their healing is huge. Please do not underestimate the importance of this. Remember, as you heal others, you are also healed. The healer often gets more healing than their partner! Good for them!

What Does Tribal Healing Have to do with Solving the Native American Dilemma? That is, being ignored by the USA corporation policy makers, which has been devastating to us/them.

I believe and teach that the healing and restoration of our American land and lost rights is linked to and re-establishing the languages, customs and societies of our Native peoples. Our respect for the Native spiritual connection with the land and with Great Spirit is essential for national healing to occur. That means that the invading Europeans need to get more spiritual and closer to the rhythms of nature and of the earth. This includes respecting the indigenous peoples that are so connected to this land. Respect is so lacking in this day and age of "profits at all costs".

Now how does one do that when the predominant European thought process is a vacuum when it comes to spiritual awareness, except for guilt and aggression? Often what they call spirituality is empty rituals, or listening to someone else's interpretation of their views of social customs or "religious doctrine."

I believe and teach that the inclusion of all our angles, saints, ancestors, guides, family members, friends, classmates, and acquaintances forms a critical mass for healing. When one thinks about that, it's a lot of beings you are healing. I call that "Your Tribe." That introduces the concept of what I call Universal Holographic Programming and healing. When you ask your tribe to ask and include their tribes into the healing, that adds power and permanence to your healing. Then when you invite every other being in the Universe to join in their and your healing, you get global, Universal healing on a huge scale. You are healing the entire field. This process needs to be introduced into church groups, clubs, family gatherings, any large gatherings, including concerts, ball games, after the games of course! And into TV programs and PBS specials. How about taking it to the United Nations, and have the U.N. members take the healing method to their tribes?

Table of Contents for Your Healing Information

Forward: Who Are We?
And Where Did We Come From?

Two Hearts Healing Center has been resolving early childhood pain and trauma since 2006 in Cupertino, California. We teach that when one thoroughly understands where pain comes from, and one has a healing system that works, it is not difficult to resolve pain. Once early childhood pain is balanced, the later negative health issues are extinguished. In other words: "Once your early childhood pain is balanced, systems in your body work better." Balance and flow is good in your body. You can balance an unbalanced system. Happy exploration and balancing healing energy for you. Balance equals flow equals health. This book has the key process for doing this.

Our Recurring Message

Our recurring message in this and all our books is that early childhood trauma, whether accidental or deliberate, compromises one's immune system, and has the potential to shorten one's life significantly as shown in The ACE Medical Study. Traumatized nerves can shut down vital body functions including rationality in the brain. There has never been a healing system that can repair this damage until this system was developed. Clients say that they have been given a new life after several sessions of two hours each. You are worth fixing regardless of the severity of your past trauma. You are not your past, and you, the being are not the pain of your past. The effects of the past damage can be fixed by balancing the stuck energy from early trauma. This is liberating news for those that suffered past trauma, and who want to free themselves from the effects of that trauma. These statements become real when you resolve to do this healing work and witness the results. We are results driven. If it doesn't work why do it, and why write books about it?

Also, instead of allowing a medical professional to fix your body when you are ill, how about being proactive about your health and take responsibility for your own health. It is okay to have such a strong immune system that most diseases can not take hold in your body. This saves you time, money and hassle.

This is serious business. One can deliberately reverse the effects of their early childhood trauma using these processes. We believe and teach that one can strengthen and improve their immune system, just like one can increase muscle strength and stamina, and increase their longevity adding healthy and happy, drug free years to their lives.

Our Last Best Solution to Resolve the Conflicts of Earth

Note: To you, the reader, The more you don't like what's in the news every day on TV, the more you need to seriously look at this Universal Resolution Programming process. It works. This is an audience participation process. We all invite our ancestors, angels, guides, saints, healers, families, friend, and loved ones. Earth needs large groups of people doing this process to cause this needed shift. We resolve global conflicts one person at a time, in groups, with their tribes joining in. This creates a huge group of participants and the energy to produce the shift. You with your tribe can be the shift you want to see in the world. At one point we collectively invite all the beings in the Universe to join the healing because they may never had an opportunity to heal, having never been asked nor invited. This process is written so the reader can understand it, to quickly learn it, to be confident enough to try it on a small group at first to test it, then to try it on larger groups. It works extremely well. It took thirty years to make it this fast and this effective. It is here for your use. Use it!

You are reminded that Albert Einstein said that; "You can't solve a problem/issue with the same mind that created it." So this is the shift in perception that changes that.

The X, Y & Z Coordinates of Universal Holographic Programming Are,

X. Whenever two or more are gathered in my name, there I will be.
Y. My people get not because they ask not… It is now okay to ask. Ask, and ask, and ask. Keep putting that intention out there. Remember, "Ask and you shall receive!" It doesn't say, "think about it for a long time and wish about it." It says, "Ask!"
Z. Your family and tribe being asked to be a part of the healing adds numbers and Power to the process. There is power in numbers. The more numbers there are the more effective is the process. Your tribe deeply wants to be a part of this earth's healing, and in being a part of your life. They need to be asked. Those are the rules.

What Makes You Think I Am Important Enough To Make A Difference In This World?

You are more than a small part of the Universal Hologram. You can make more than a small impact on this shift. There are only a few rotten apples on this earth and this process puts them in an agreeable mood. Just because you were told you can't make a difference does not make it true. You are far more powerful than anyone ever told you. You can use this process to create the shift you desire. The more you do it the faster the shift occurs. This is the only group healing process that heals whole groups at a time. It works and it is here for your use. Do it! Take the ball and run with it!

The Axioms of Holographic Programming

1. You must first give before you can expect to receive.
2. This process provides that offering of a gift from you.
3. The gifts of the Universe come to you through people. That's why including them in your healing works so well. You get a session and others heal along with you.
4. One can do selfish healing of only yourself, but why would you not want to include your tribe? They need healing, too. And it requires so little effort from you.
5. You heal the Hologram with your vision and with your intention to heal it.
6. When you add all of your tribe to this intention and vision of healing, it goes viral very quickly. You want the maximum amount of healing for the maximum amount of beings, with the minimum amount of time spent. Never underestimate this multiplier effect of asking your tribe and other beings for help, because this is huge.
7. Let's say you have ten angels, one hundred ancestors, ten family members, and ten friends and you invite them to join your intention and vision for the hologram to shift.
8. You ask all of them to bring all of their friends, and their tribes, you now have a huge gathering of beings joining you.
9. Then you ask all these newcomers to bring all of their friends, and their tribes. This quickly could become millions of members. The more the better.
10. Now, you're going to ask all the people that have ever lived to be a part of this healing, all the angels that have ever been created, every saint and holy person,

every pet and animal that has ever existed, every being that has not been included, and anyone else you can think of.

11. This is because we heal as a tribe, and we all need healing, and we heal all together.

12. Here's the key, "You don't have to know them to invite them." They just need to be asked to join the healing. You may be the first and only one to ask them. They may be very grateful for that, and they may reward you for the favor.

13. A beings greatest fear is to be forgotten. This process asks them to come forward and to join in and to be healed. There are prossibly more beings on the other side than there are here on earth.

14. Now, you're going to ask out loud to get their agreement to join in and help you.

15. When you ask, you also visualize your intention, for this change on earth as if it has already happened…

16. You say out loud, "My constant intention is that there is a permanent shift in global social consciousness from fear and conflict to understanding, compassion and resolution, no matter what it takes."

17. You now have the "100ᵗʰ Monkey" energetically happening, see page 20 for the story, and that is about one tenth of one percent of the Universal Hologram.

18. When you join a group of beings working and aligning for the same goal, well…

19. This is not an instant process, It requires reaching the critical mass of participants.
    That number has not been reached as of today, but with your help it is possible.

20. It is okay to ask incessantly of yourself and your tribe, as a daily mantra. "Compassion, harmony, resolution, healing." Out loud of course. And get your tribe and all beings to do the same.

21. Please join me on this quest. When we reach the "100ᵗʰ Monkey" everything will shift.

22. Is it possible that the terrorists on earth will never figure out what happened to their destructive plans!

Earth has angels and guides, too, just like you and I. Those angels and guides want the paradigm of earth to shift from international strife to never-ending peace, harmony and balance so that the healing of the societies of Earth can take place.

This is part of the plan for transformation which is happening on earth. All the great spiritual leaders from the past have returned to be a part of this transformation. When asked why they would come back they said, "We would not miss this event for the world!" They also said that everyone on earth is here for this transformation weather they are aware of it or not.

This is the key to this planetary holographic programming. Because when we consciously do this programming, we are assisted by the earth's angels and guides. This gives the process a quantum boost over what we can do ourselves alone. When the tiniest part of the hologram shifts, the entire hologram changes. The paradigm shift is part of this hologram. I believe your individual identity, DNA is part of this hologram. Each of you are a big part of this individual identity.

1. When enough parts of the hologram ask for change, the change takes place.
2. You, just as you are, are more than a small part of this hologram. That means you have the power to make this change. Just think of the possibilities...
3. Gather mentally before you, your ancestors, your present extended family and friends, your angels, guides, masters, and your church congregations, community groups, include the people of your neighborhood, county, state and nation. Call this "Your Gathering," or "Your Tribe." I prefer "Tribe."
4. Getting help from Earth's angels and guides can't possibly hurt. Ask them now to join your group.
5. Thank them out loud for being a part of this request. And ask all of them out loud to join you to be part of this holographic shift process.
6. It is okay to tell them out loud why this shift is so important.
7. Remember that taking massive action trumps wishful thinking.
8. Remember that in asking out loud, one receives, and that, "Whenever two or more are gathered there I will be." There is a synergy to a group.
9. Tell your gathering out loud for a second time why it is so important for you to shift this paradigm. Getting help from Earth's angels and guides can't possibly hurt.
10. Remember that some or all your tribe is related to other people's tribes. This where it goes viral on the holographic energy plane! Wow!
11. This is global programming goes way beyond prayer or wishful thinking, or complaining as far as effectiveness goes.
12. Then say out loud, "I want unconditional world peace right now."
13. Say out loud, "I want unconditional conflict resolution right now."
14. "I want unconditional interpersonal harmony right now.

15. "I want the Universal hologram to reprogram right now for this harmony, world peace and conflict resolution. Now! And so it is, and so it is done."
16. Proclaim it out loud! "I want it now!"
17. "I want unconditional world peace, friendship and harmony right now."
18. Say out loud, "I want unconditional world unity right now."
19. "To all my tribes and their tribes, go ahead and add your own intentions for healing here."
20. The people of earth are transformed from greed and fear to respect for all life, respect for each other, and respect for the earth.
21. Add your own wishes here.

Can you imagine the power of doing this process in a stadium of 50,000 people inviting all of their family gatherings? At this level we definitely share tribal members.

Holograms

A hologram projects a 3-D image. Hologram might be the wrong word to use for the Universal thought image that we are. We are part of that 3-D thought image. That's why I am calling it the hologram. It's that energetic connection with things unseen, but powerfully influential.

It's Never Too Late to Improve Your Health

It' never too late to improve your immune system, your health and longevity. Even if you are ninety-eight years old, if you are determined, you can do these processes and make a significant conscious difference in your health.

How to Do the Heart to Heart Healing Process

It is so important to your health to balance stuck energy in your heart area. You can heal stuck trauma from the past and this frees you to lead a life in present time. Recent medical studies suggest that one's life and health improves with energy balance. This is a two person hands-on-healing process. You sit at right angles to each other and the process runs from five minutes up to a half-hour. The giver is patiently holding the heart area of the receiver. Place one hand on the front heart and one hand on the back heart. One can do this process watching TV, waiting for food to arrive at a restaurant, or most any other places. The giver may say "Heal," or "Heal now," or "I love you," or "Peace be still (to the random energy, not to the heart)," or "I'm quieting and balancing random, non-productive heart energy." It feels as if the giver is gently holding a small animal or a small bird in their hands. Your heart is sacred energy. Your hands are healing energy. Your partner will say, "Your hands feel so good." That's energy balancing. Keep doing the process.

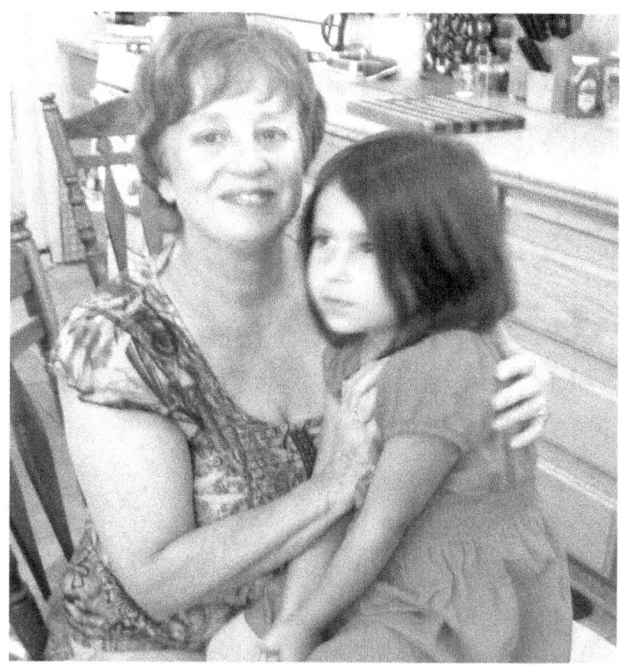

Heart Healing a Grandchild

It may feel as if the giver is holding a small animal or a small bird in their hands. The focus is to bring calm to random heart energy. The giver is steadying-quieting random, non-productive heart energy.

Why Work on the Heart Area?

You are made of love. That love resides in your heart. This is ancient wisdom. The heart is the largest-strongest energy in the body. When the healer balances the random, unaligned energy, the "calm" circulates throughout the body to all points where the blood flows. Quieting trauma in the body's largest energy source has huge beneficial healing rewards. The process looks simple, it runs deep and the gains can be huge, even if one feels nothing. This is not a "feel" process. This is a heal process. One is better off when there is balance and flow in the body. Balance is healing. Stuck energy can cause illness. This process is not just done once. A half an hour session should be done once or twice a day for a week to start. Anyone interested in improving the health of another can learn to do these processes and get a result. It just takes the determination to learn the process, practice it to become proficient, and then doing it with a lot of people to get the feel of it. Once the skill is learned it stays forever.

In severe cases it may take months of work but you and your loved ones are worth the time and the work. Remember as they heal, you also heal. It's tribal energy healing, and it works because we share our tribe's energy. One's belief system is not a part of this healing. To start learning, just meet with friends and start doing the process. We all need healing. Your entire tribe needs healing whether you believe it or not. Work on as many as you can.

Starting on page 52, there is an expanded version of this process. Both versions work equally well. This one is easy to do in public, like waiting for food to arrive at a restaurant.

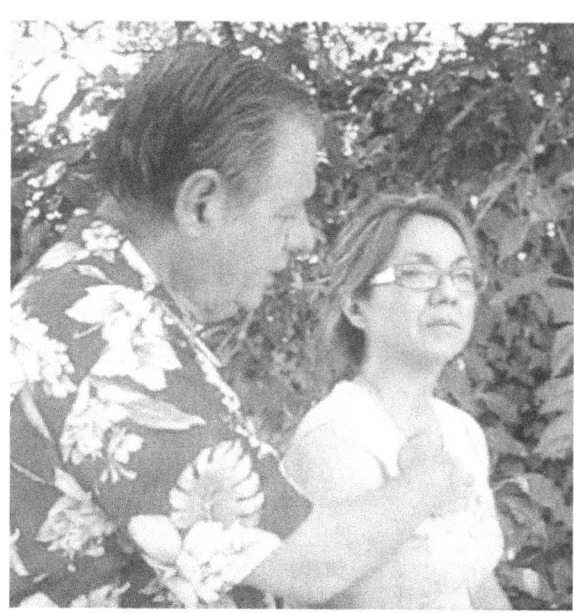

Heart Healing an Adult

How Does One Know When They Are Done?

Note: This is a breakthrough in the field of healing. As a test has never existed to show when one is done!

Great Question: With a little practice one can feel the balance. Imbalance presents itself with uneven warmness or coolness from the front to the back of the heart area. One may feel one area increase in heat or coolness upon first touching. That shows imbalance. The real skill here is noticing that the heat or coolness changes and increases and decreases. One is done in that session when the temperature does not change over several minutes. This can take awhile to get to this point. The first few sessions should be five to fifteen minutes to start. When one first starts, one might feel they are done when the first cycle of change completes. One is not done yet. It is better to overdo the process than to leave stuck energy in place. Unbalanced energy is stuck, and stuck energy compromises one's health. There is a medical study that validates this fact, **"The ACE Study,"** by Kaiser Permanente, Google and read it! This healing process is as important as good nutrition, deep breathing, sleep and exercise. It's that important to your health and well being. This process can bring people out of comas, so don't take it lightly, it runs deep. Thank you. This process works miraculously well on animals, too, dogs, cats, horses, and all as their nervous systems are similar to ours.

In an occupation where one can not touch their clients nor children, have the children or clients work on each other. People are willing to help each other, and this will change group dynamics.

How Can I Tell If My Present Healing Method Is Working, That Is, "Resolving" All The Stuck Energy?

This Heart Healing Process can test other modalities for their effectiveness. This is a breakthrough in the field of healing. As a test has never existed to test other healing methods for "doneness!" One can "check" for completeness. Thank God there is a way to test other healing methods to see if they got all the stuck energy. Stuck energy equals illness, and flowing energy is healing energy. To test a healing method one sits or stands at right angles to their partner and does the Heart Healing Process for several minutes. Be aware upon first touching the front heart and back heart of any rising heat at the instant of touching. Please be aware that the heat can rise so quickly that it feels like they are just naturally warm or "hot." Then see if the heat increases or decreases. Any change in the heat indicates there is more work to be done. Then you can give your partner the gift right there of working on them to balance the stuck energy. You and yours need the best chance for survival. This process gives you that healthy edge.

Check for Completeness of the Healing

This is not a judgment of other modalities, this is a tool to check for completeness. One places one hand on the front heart and one hand on the back heart and patiently waits to see if the energy rises or falls, heats up or cools down. Any fluctuation or difference in heat or coolness indicates there is energy there that needs to be balanced. Balance is good. Knowing one is complete is a gift and a blessing. This method provides that confidence. Happy learning, happy balancing, and happy healing. We believe with this method we can start to heal the world. It's worth the work. It is a worthy goal. This author does not write anything that does not work extremely well.

Note: This method is about healing your heart, and the hearts past and present of your tribes and peoples. We need not go into all the horrible atrocities the Europeans have committed against our original indigenous American Peoples. When the Europeans arrived here there were one hundred million Native Americans. Now there are just a handful left. Did you know that every treaty that has ever been signed between the U.S. Government corporation (Europeans) and the Native tribes has been broken many times over? And you wonder why they had to kill off most of our indigenous population? This book is not a political nor a social statement nor a rant. It is a workable path to restoring wholeness. Wholeness is healing. Respect is balance and healing.

Would You Benefit from this Healing Technique?

1. Have you ever fallen more than three feet to the ground? Or have you had other severe falls, like down stairs, out of trees, off roofs, off fences, off cliffs, off horses, off ladders, off bicycles, trips and falls?
2. Have you ever been hit in the head with a ball, rock, or other hard object, even if accidentally while playing sports?
3. Have you ever played football or other sports where head injuries can happen?
4. Have you ever been hit by a baseball bat or hockey stick to the head or body, even if accidental?
5. Have you already had a stroke, heart attack, cancer, etc. where your life was threatened?* (*Important Note: There is no representation here that this process can fix these issues. The damage is done. This process can balance stuck energy associated with these events.)
6. Have you ever been severely beaten, or beaten up?
7. Have you ever had broken bones or painful surgeries?
8. Have you ever been in an auto, boat, plane, or train accident/crash?
9. Have you ever been bitten hard by an animal, person or bird?
10. Have you ever been confined for long periods of time?
11. Have you experienced any abuse as a child sexually, or otherwise?
12. Have you ever been enslaved, starved, tied up and punished, drugged, shunned or emotionally abused?
13. Have you ever been alcoholic or addicted to drugs for more than 3 months?
14. Have you ever had a bad drug trip? Overdose, etc.?
15. Have you ever been shot or shot at or tased?
16. Have you ever been in a combat zone as a soldier or as a civilian? PTSD?
17. Have you ever had a life altering trauma, emotional or physical?
18. Have you ever had nerve issues or disorders, like neuropathy - numbness?
19. Have you ever been in a coma? How about blackouts?
20. Do you suffer from chronic pain in any part of your body?
21. Are you on pain medication?
22. Do you suffer from unexplained pain?
23. Do parts of your body creek or hurt when you get up in the morning? How about shooting pains? Charlie horses?
24. Have you ever lied to your doctor about having pain, or other conditions?
25. Have you ever been told: "Your pain is all in your head?" Or: "You just have to live with it."

26. Do you suffer from unexplainable chronic life conditions?
27. Do you avoid people at all costs?
28. Are you alone in a crowd?
29. Do you have few or no friends?
30. Are you depressed most of the time?
31. Do you have no interest in life?
32. Do you make more than three mistakes a day?
33. Do you hate your life, or resent your being born, or having been victimized?
34. Does everything you touch "turn to crap?"

If you answered "Yes" to any three or more of these questions then you could possibly benefit from doing this healing method, that is after you discuss these issues with a qualified medical professional and you get help. This method balances early cellular memories of pain/trauma.

Huge healing issues can resolve with this method. It's worth the price of this book and it's worth the effort to learn and to do this method. You are worth the time. You are worth the effort. And you are worth the healing. This method can not hurt, and it can only help. It's like vitamins, if you don't need them you feel nothing, and if you do need them they are like miracle, life-changing supplements.

You and your loved ones are worth the relief.

Note: These front pages are laid out for effective display on Amazon's web site. These are the core messages of this book presented here. My hope is to spark interest in healing chronic pain, especially persistent psycho-somatic pain rooted in early childhood trauma.

Q. People ask me, "Why would you write another book on healing? Aren't their enough books already?"

No! In a bookstore with ten-thousand different books on healing, this is the only one that makes your body's energy system and healing easy to understand, easy to do, and where one can study it in one day, do the method as it is taught, and see a result that same day.* That has not existed before this book and this method. In this world where everything seems to be instant. This method is as close to instant as one can get. You are worth the results. You are worth being healthy. Your loved ones are worth the results and the increased health. The processes in this book are worth your serious consideration, time and effort.

Are the Results Worth the Time it Takes?

A: The real question is, "Are you, your loved ones, and your tribe worth the time it takes to heal the pain of the past?" It is possible to neutralize the effects of past trauma. Our message here is that you are enough, and your partner is enough. That combined "enough-ness" plus your willingness to work for a dramatic change in health equals better health for you and your whole tribe.

After her first two hour session, a lady named Joan called the next day and said: "I am no longer depressed. And projects that I put on the back-burner ten years ago are coming to life, and I am starting to accomplish what I was born on this planet to do." At the end of that session she said, "Well that was a nice massage." Meaning, "No big deal." **Note:** The results often "just show up later" and surprise the participants. The positive gains are definitely worth the work.

Authors Note: I firmly believe that results like this are worth the work and time it takes to get a result. Especially when one knows that we are energetically connected and healing of one helps heal the whole. It is okay to help heal the world, one healing session at a time. In other books there are processes that heal whole groups.

There is a point where we as a society will realize that we are spiritual beings living a physical existence, and at that time we will make laws supporting that idea, and we will treat each other as such. I patiently await that day.

Every day I sit at my computer and ask, "Why Me? Why did you pick me for this work?" And they say, "Why NOT you?"

The State of the Healing Arts

Q. So What Makes Your Healing Method Different and Special, and Why Should I Care?

A. Even with the tremendous medical breakthroughs made each year, one has to wonder how and why the original source of the illness is not found nor addressed. This book is the first accurate proven method that eliminates the cause of the present pain, which is the unbalanced, stuck early childhood trauma. Trauma causes life energy to get stuck. It remains stuck until it is balanced. I have worked on eighty year olds that had all the original stuck energy intact, even decades later. Once balanced, the stuck energy can not return. The proof of this healing is the detox reaction one can go through in addition to the softening of facial features of your partner. This method is certainly better than pushing pills and surgeries as the final remedy to chronic pain. The greatest shock is the news that there can be a healing method that actually balances stuck energy and thus can heal. There is no intention to disrespect pills nor drugs because, if they are critically needed, they are life saving miracle drugs. It is the over medicating or promoting that pills and surgeries are the only remedy to chronic pain that we take issue with. This healing method provides a spiritual remedy to the basic cause of the pain. There is tremendous wisdom in this book. Read it and understand it, and do it, and reap the benefits for you and your loved ones. This method works extremely well and it is worth your serious consideration, trial, proof and mastery.

You Can Rapidly Heal Yourself and Your Loved Ones

Your health is important. We all need a health improvement method that works well. You can choose to increase your own health potential and that of loved ones. This method has not been available before now. This method is presented here in a highly learnable form so it's easy to understand and to do. Medical studies have shown that early childhood trauma can shorten ones life, and cause other difficulties, especially if one had a lot of trauma. You can choose to balance the stuck energy of early trauma and improve your chances for better health. You can also choose to improve your loved ones chances for better health. This is so real and so doable. This method is worth your consideration and your effort to master it. The rewards go far beyond the effort it takes. Anyone committed to making a difference in the lives of others can learn and master this process and actually make a difference.

This method and processes are not an instant action. It may require many sessions. You and your loved ones are worth the time, the love and the effort. It is difficult to do these processes with people you do not care about. The more one cares the more effective the work becomes. There can be a healing energy to past and present relationship connections. This is worth exploring.

Note: I have met married couples who never thought of asking their partner about early childhood trauma. Now there is a remedy. The early unbalanced trauma is like unhandled clutter in your house. A word to the wise. You can now fix this situation.

Youtube Videos that you can watch online:

Youtube Video #1 by Paul Barbaro: http://www.youtube.com/watch?v=M_CdVe-_qsY

Youtube Video #2: http://www.youtube.com/watch?v=FE-aNtbuqlk

Youtube Video #3: http://www.youtube.com/watch?v=XunCrduVOto

On Youtube.com one can type in: **"Barbaro – Healing"** and watch any new videos that we post.

Editors Note: One can also see **FREE** training videos of this technique at www.healingangelguides.com/   Please click on "Training" and watch these videos with a friend or partner, read this book together and then take turns doing this process on each other. One can get a result while doing the exercises taught in these videos. The gains can be tremendous.

Please do not discount the effectiveness of these processes before giving them a fair trial. They work very well. In our office we have seen chronic pain go from an "8" on a scale from one to ten, ten being severe pain, from an "8" to a "2" in two hours time, and the pain did not increase from a "2" within a two year period of time. We can't say it is permanent, but two years is a long time to have less pain.

Other Books by Paul Barbaro

Healing Our Community – Real Healing for our communities and for our nation. Hundreds can be healed in minutes. And may they never be the same, and better. **ISBN-13: 978-1495281457**

Angelology – A Better Connection with Universal Mind. Invite your Angels, Ancestors and Tribe to heal with you. This Book has helpful natural ways to Increase Immunity and Health. **ISBN-13: 978-1496132178**

Resolving Global Conflicts - When You're Ready for the Shift in 2016! Global Healing for the masses. This book contains a group process to speed up healing on this planet. **ISBN-13:978-1523864607**

Heart to Heart Healing - When You Care Enough to Make a Difference in the Health of a Loved One. Training and a healing process to help bring balance to loved one's compromised immune systems. Helps to extend life, health, and longevity. **ISBN-13: 978-1495379369**

The Lightbearer's Handbook – Let Your Healing Light Shine Brighter. Out of print, but soon to be updated and published.

Disclaimer

based solely on the content of this publication. The information and opinions provided herein are believed to be accurate and sound at the time of publication, based on the best judgment available to the author. However, readers who rely on information in this publication to replace the advice of health care professionals, or who fail to consult with health care professionals, assume all risks of such conduct. The publisher and author is/are not responsible for errors or omissions.

These statements have not been evaluated by the Food and Drug Administration. This product or process is not intended to diagnose, treat, cure, or prevent any disease.

If one has pain then one is advised to see a medical professional immediately. If one is under a doctor's care, one must get their doctor's permission to receive these energy healing processes. Pain is symptomatic. Always seek medical advice from your physician or other qualified healthcare provider for any questions one may have regarding any medical condition including pain. And under no

circumstances discontinue taking any prescribed medications without your doctor's permission. There are life threatening major diseases and medical conditions that have no symptoms at all. Regularly scheduled medical checkups are extremely valuable.

When you body is under attack by bacteria or viruses, they take over and have an energy and life of their own. There is nothing in this healing method that kills bacteria nor viruses. Nor is there anything in this method that replaces lost bone, cartilage, organs, brain cells, or any body parts that have atrophied or died. This method can not do anything to remedy a pinched nerve nor a condition of a physical malfunction that causes present pain. Nor can it do anything for terminal people in the process of dying. Please see your medical doctor or professional when you are under viral or bacterial attack. This book teaches an ancient traditional spiritual healing method modernized, brought into the Twenty-First century, and made easy to learn and to do. People who wish to try or do this energy balancing technique do so at their own peril. This is a spiritual healing method. It is strongly advised to do this healing work under a religious minister or under the care of a medical doctor or health professional.

More Disclaimer: I, Paul Barbaro, created this spiritual work and it is a complement to conventional medicine and alternative healing methods. I'm a minister and this spiritual energy work is not a substitute for conventional medical treatment of any kind, physical or psychological. For such issues you should seek the proper licensed physician or qualified health care professional. This energy work may help the bio-field to come into energetic balance. Qigong theory believes when one's energy field is in balance, the body's latent healing ability can heal itself. I can make no promises nor guarantees about the results of this work. I am very grateful for this opportunity to work with everyone interested in healing. I, Paul Barbaro, make absolutely no promises, no claims because every body is different and everybody responds differently to healing energy. "Viva la difference."

Revival of Ancient Traditional
"Hands on Healing" Method

One thousand years ago when someone was sick they would go to the village square. The people of the village would form a circle around the sick person and place their hands on the person for half an hour or more. The person who was sick would get better. In this tradition healing is a tribal community event. They understood that we heal together as a group.

Notice: This healing method was taught to me by two First Nation - Native American Indians in 2008. It was extensively tested on hundreds of individuals and found to be highly effective in discharging and balancing stuck energy from early childhood trauma. This healing method revives the ancient and traditional "hands-on healing" as spoken of in the Jewish sacred writings and in the Christian Bible, and uses the Buddhist, Hindu, Vedic, and Judeo-Christian teachings and upon the religious teachings of: "Do unto others as you would have them do unto you." It is also based on Chinese Tai-Chi, the movement of energy, and on Qigong, and other Asian and First American Nation (American Indian) energy religious and spiritual practices. Heart to Heart Healing University, Cupertino, California, is an ecclesiastic* educational association organized under the authority of the First Amendment of the Original Constitution for the United States, of the year of Our Lord 1789. This University is religious, it is a church university, and these healing processes are religious because they resolve spiritual stuck energy as well as the cellular memory of early physical trauma. Whatever the original intention of the Founding Fathers was for our liberty, and especially all my First Amendment Rights are asserted, reserved, and protected herewith by this Notice, claim, assertion, proclamation, and publication. The University is non-medical, non-denominational, and non-political. It is open to all races, creeds and religions, as well as to all sexual orientations. This healing center is not discriminatory nor exclusive. This is because we all can use some healing. Our ultimate hope and goal is to shift global consciousness so that we humans choose to survive at a higher level by caring for and respecting our environment, other people, ourselves, and our bodies enough to take personal responsibility for these, and to work for different outcomes than we have settled for in the past.

Note: These processes are not instant. There are no magic bullets. There are no magic pills. Your work with these processes and with your loved ones has a huge payoff off for you, for your loved ones and for your tribe for getting healthier. You and they are worth the work.

As Rome was not built in a day, and as your early trauma did not happen instantly, and as your immune system was not instantly compromised, so these processes take time and work to achieve long lasting results. You and your partner are worth the work. You both are worth the time spent, and you are both worth working toward the results. Practice, patience, and persistence does make perfect in healing work.

No claims of results can ever be made from these processes because every body and every trauma is different, and heals differently. Some chronic pain does not respond to balanced energy, one is always free to explore other avenues of healing.

Just for clarity, there is no suggestion that there is anything wrong with the reader, their families nor friends, nor any of our societies. We are all made perfectly. There is nothing wrong with you or anyone or anything else. To judge this would be an injustice to the judged. My goal is to help "Turn up your 'Light' just a little brighter." Not that it's dim. Thank you for your understanding. There is some redundancy in the writing for emphasis and used as a teaching and memory tool. There is no intent to be pedantic nor disrespectful.

This Healing Method is Not Based On Anyone's Belief System

This healing method and these processes are not based on the belief systems of either the giver nor the receiver. This healing method operates at the cellular level. It can repair damaged nerve connections at the cellular level. It can repair/forgive past ancestor's health issues. Past DNA programming can be changed.* This is good news for the pain sufferer. Recent scientific discoveries have proven that DNA and past cell trauma can be successfully be reprogrammed. This healing can bring relief to the sufferer. There is hope.

*Please see the book "The Biology of Belief" by Bruce Lipton

Native American Photos

Throughout this book there are pictures of Native Americans long past. They are blessed and honored here for their efforts to preserve their lands and their way of life. Please take time to notice the intensity of their resolve. We should never forget that they were here first before the Europeans ever set foot in America. And that there is a blessing to living in harmony with the land and with the Universe as they did.

Many of these photos are available on Pintrest, Ebay, Amazon, or Google them. Many of the photos were taken by John C. H. Grabill, and by Edward S. Curtis. Both were American ethnologists and photographers of the American West and of Native American peoples. We are extremely thankful for their work to preserve images of these Natives. This author believes that all these pictures are in the public domain. Please correct him if this is in error. Some of the pictures don't have captions. Please, if you can identify any of the tribes or people, that information would be a great help. Feel free to send us your thoughts.

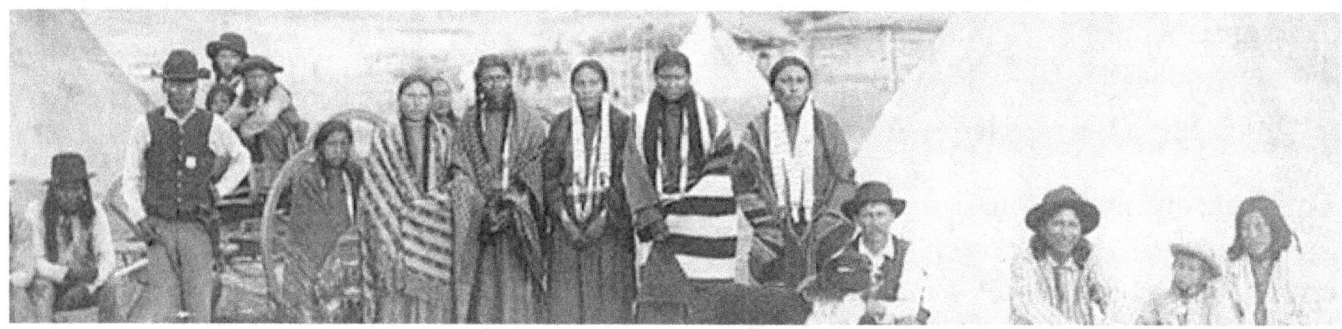

The Indian Girl's Home. John C. H. Grabill, 1890.

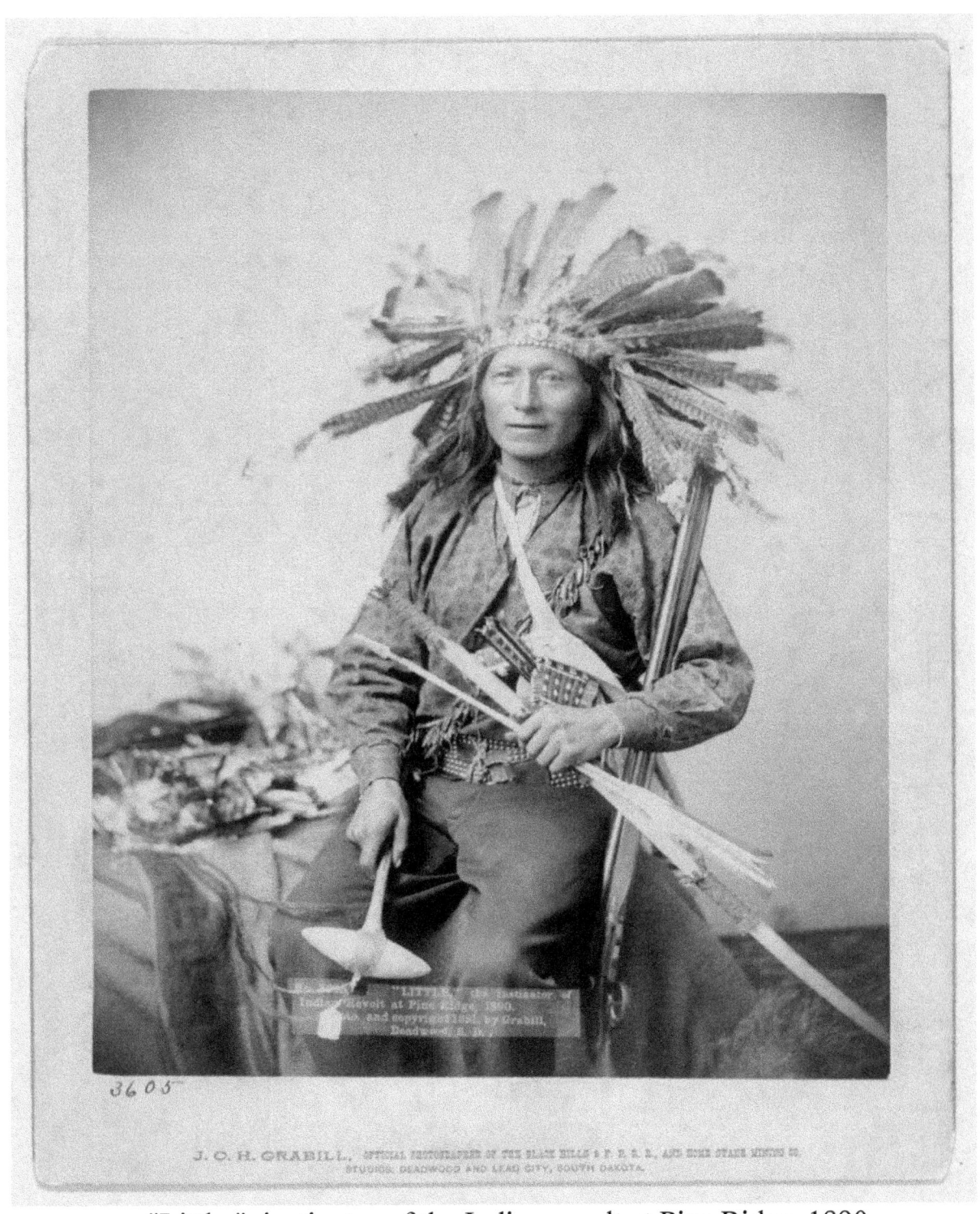

"Little," instigator of the Indian revolt at Pine Ridge, 1890.
- John C. H. Grabill, photographer. www.liveinternet.ru

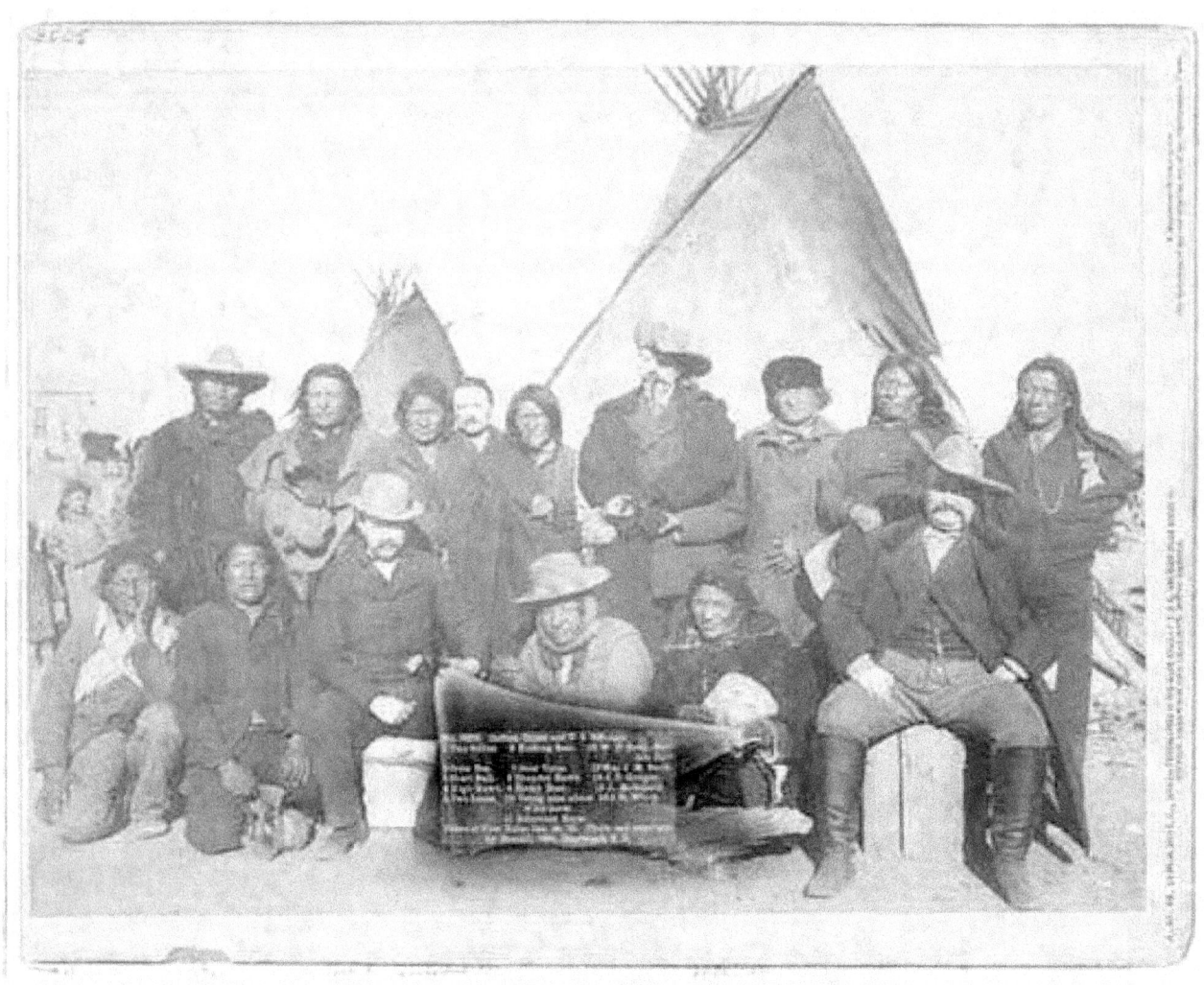

Short Bull, Kicking Bear, Good Voice, Young Man Afraid, American Horse as
reference. American-Tribes.com

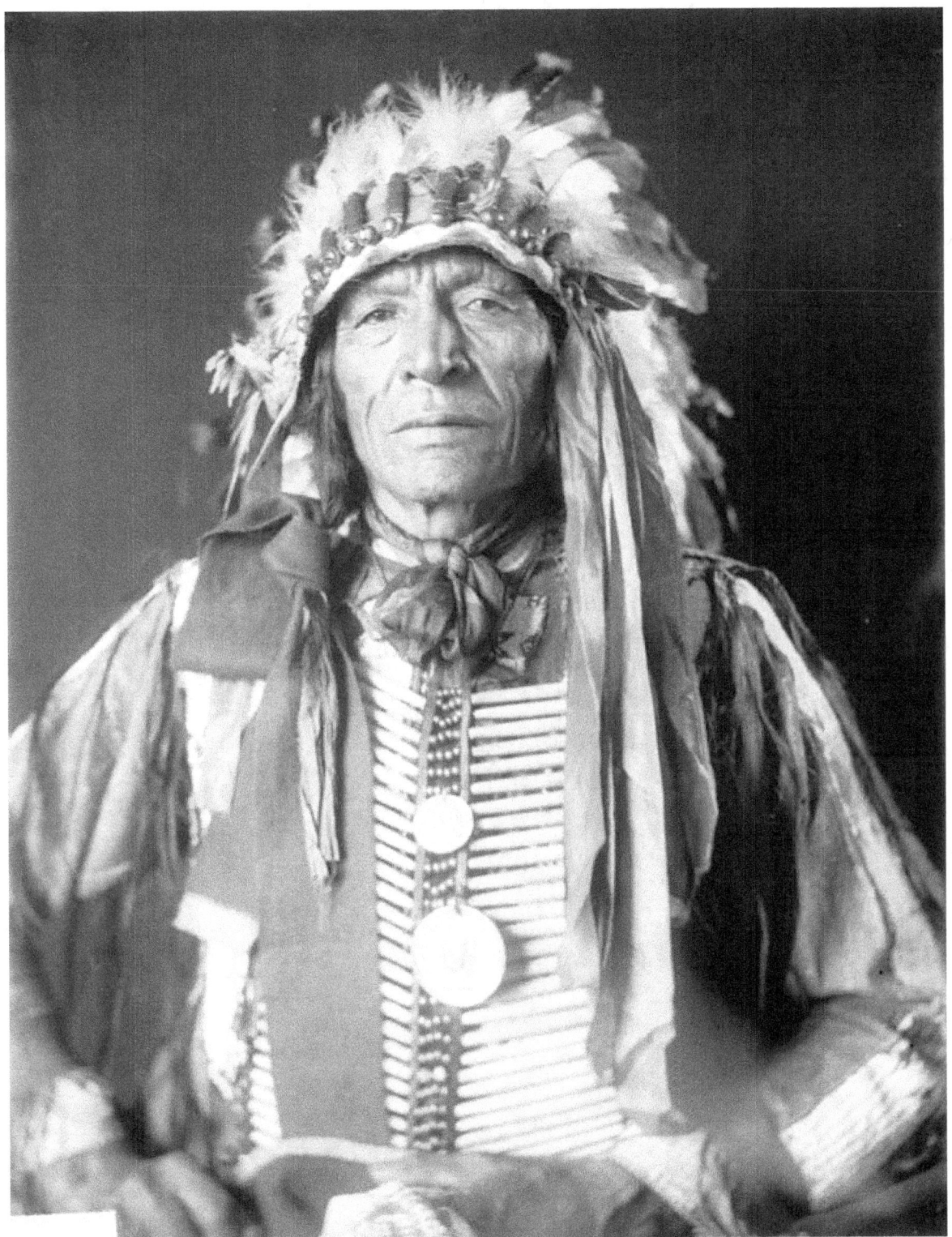

High Pipe, 1909   http://amertribes.proboards.com/thread/1302/post-wounded-knee-photo-again#ixzz3tQNLjlTo

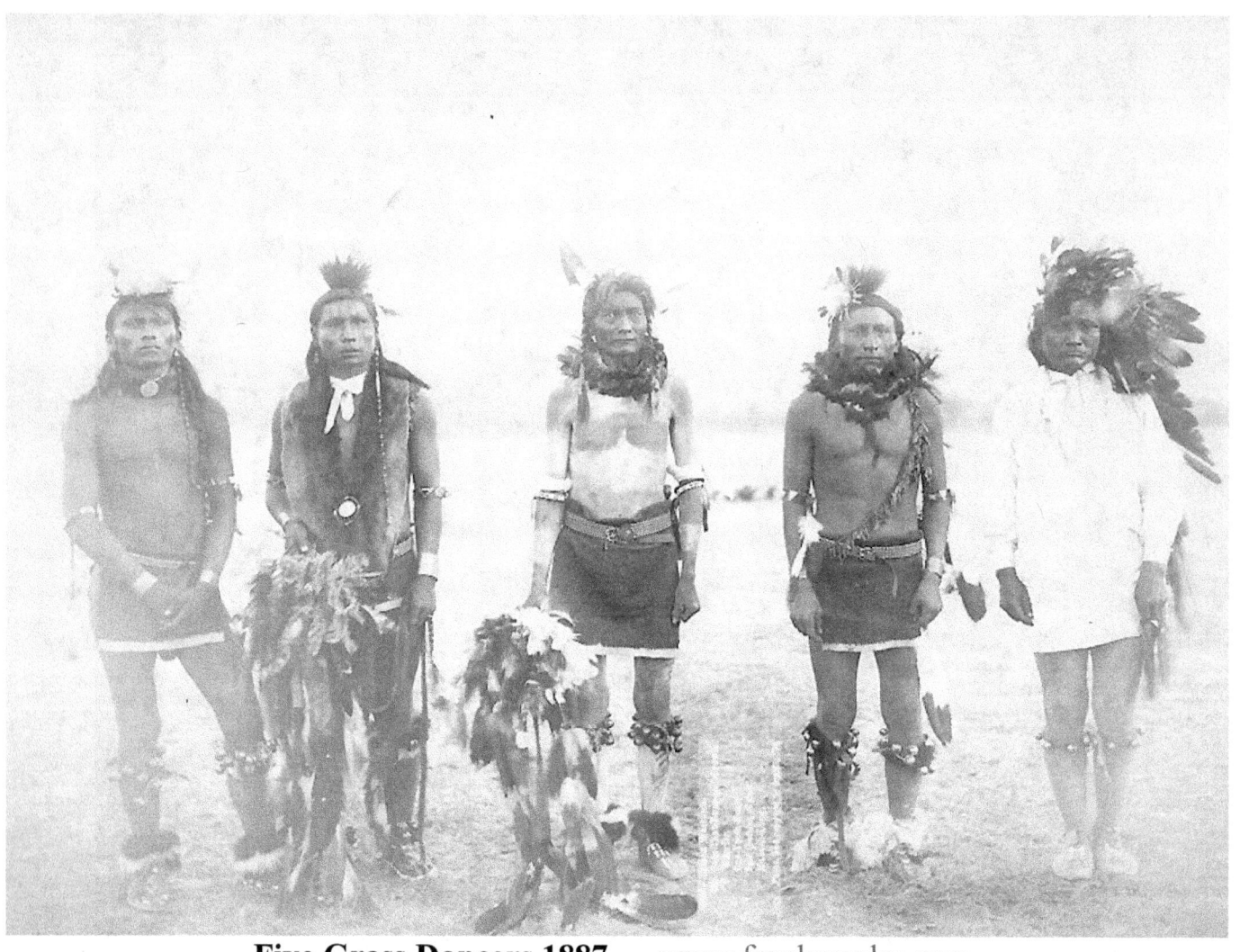

Five Grass Dancers 1887,
Dance on the Cheyenne River, S.D.-on or near Cheyenne River Reservation 1890.
Indian Warriors = Bear-that-Runs-and-Growls, Warrior, One-Tooth-Gone, Sole
(bottom of foot), Make-it-Long. Photo: John C. H. Grabill.

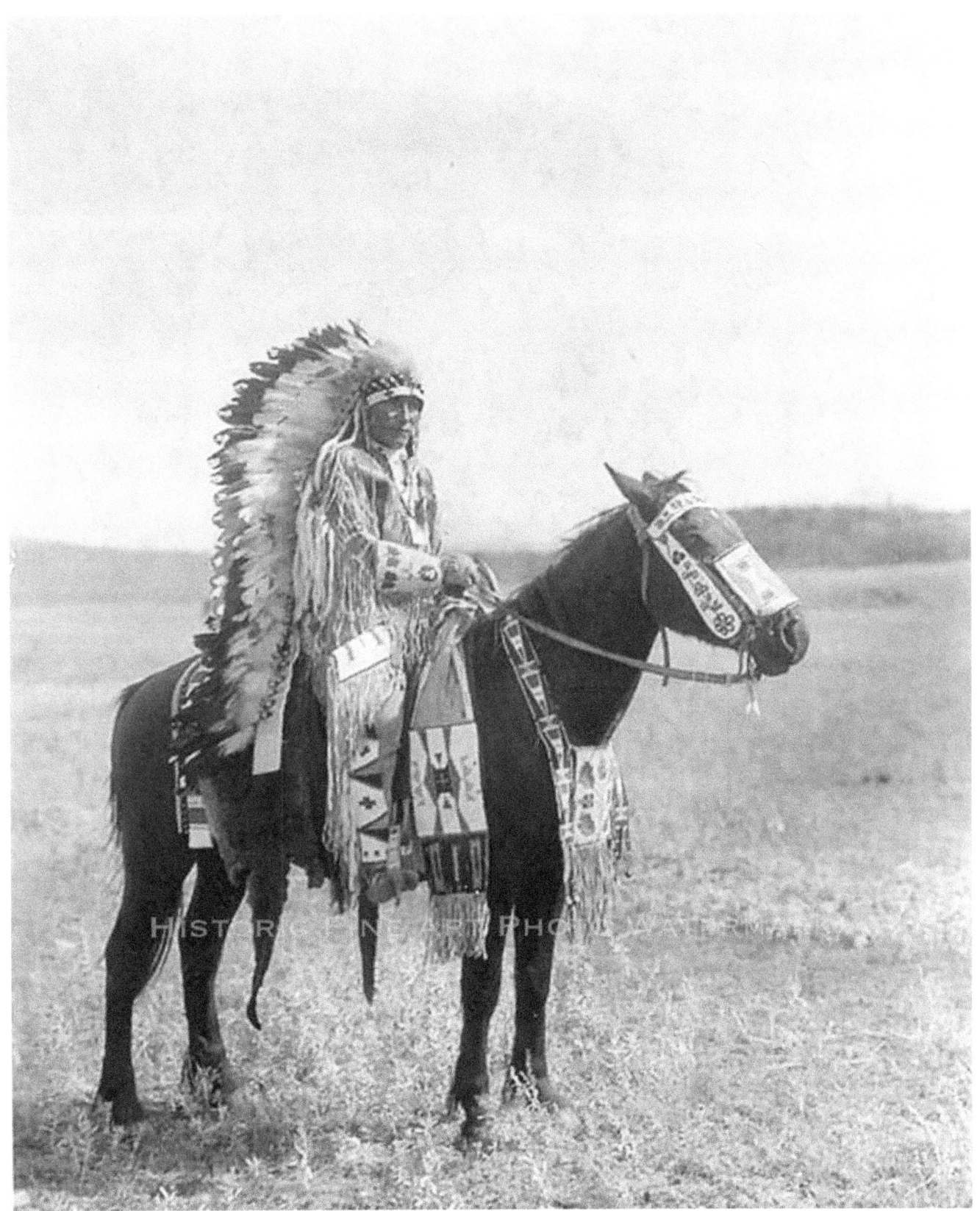

xli

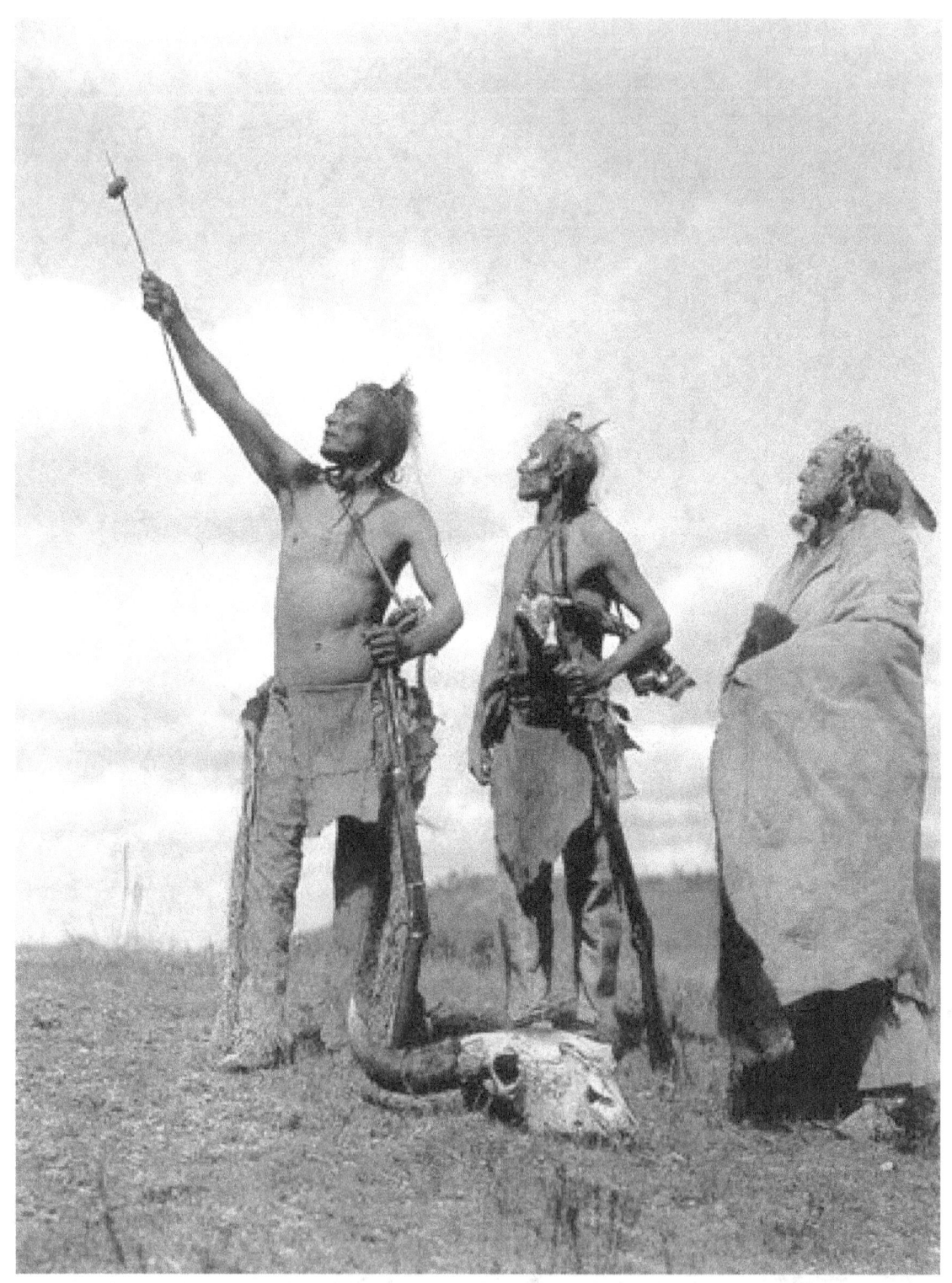

The Oath

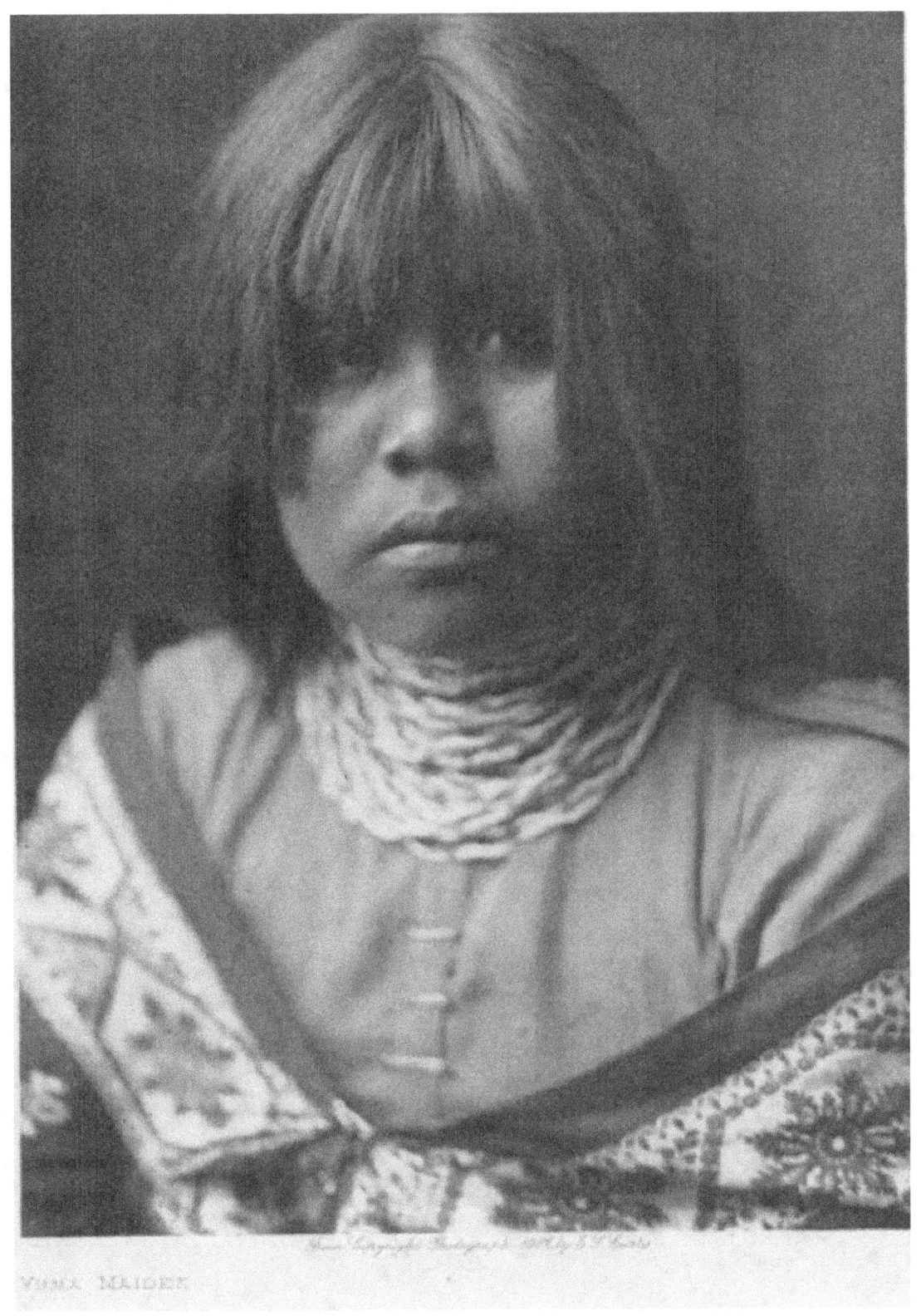

YUMA MAIDEN

From Copyright Photograph 1907 by E. S. Curtis

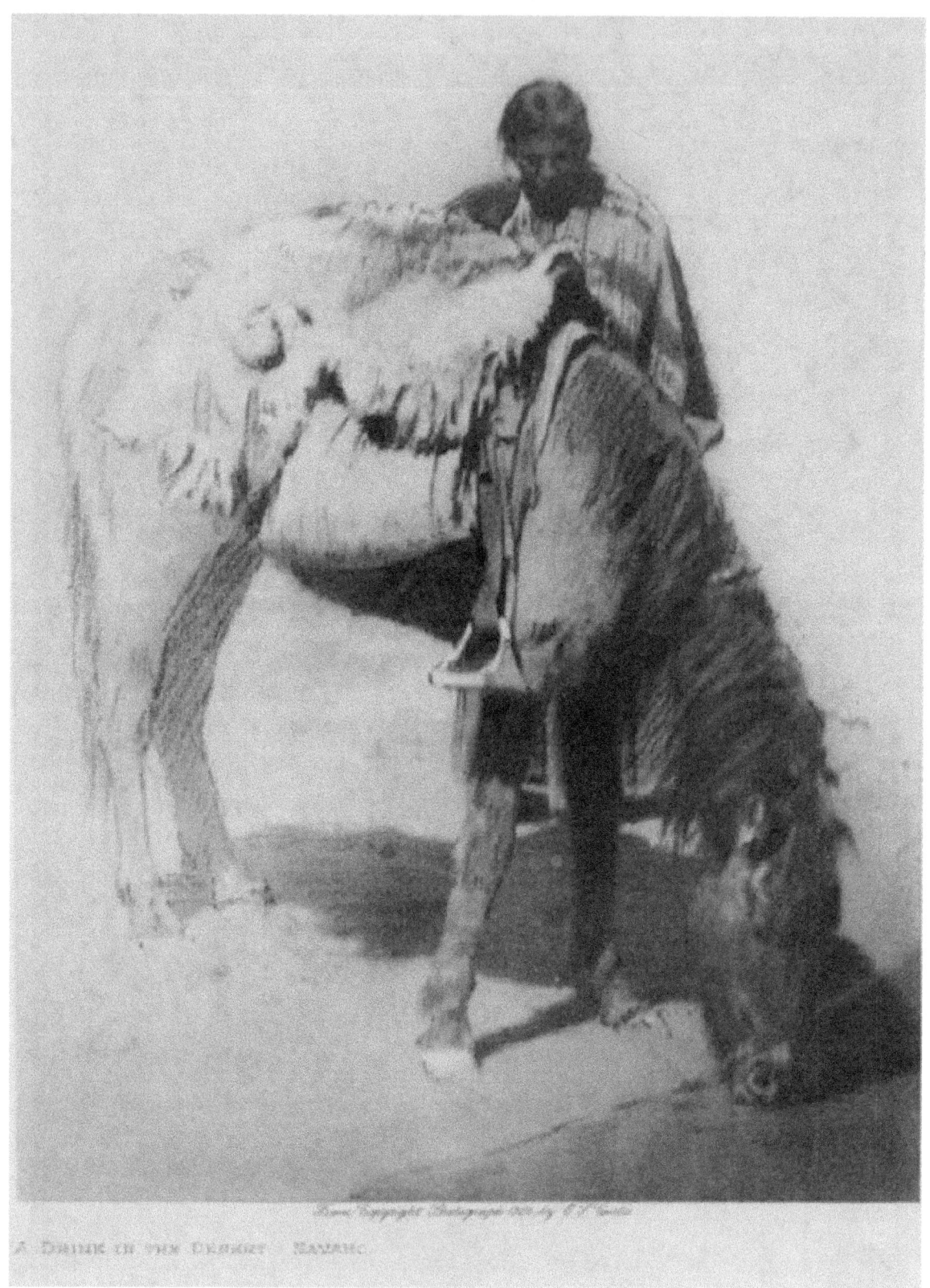

A DRINK IN THE DESERT   NAVAHO

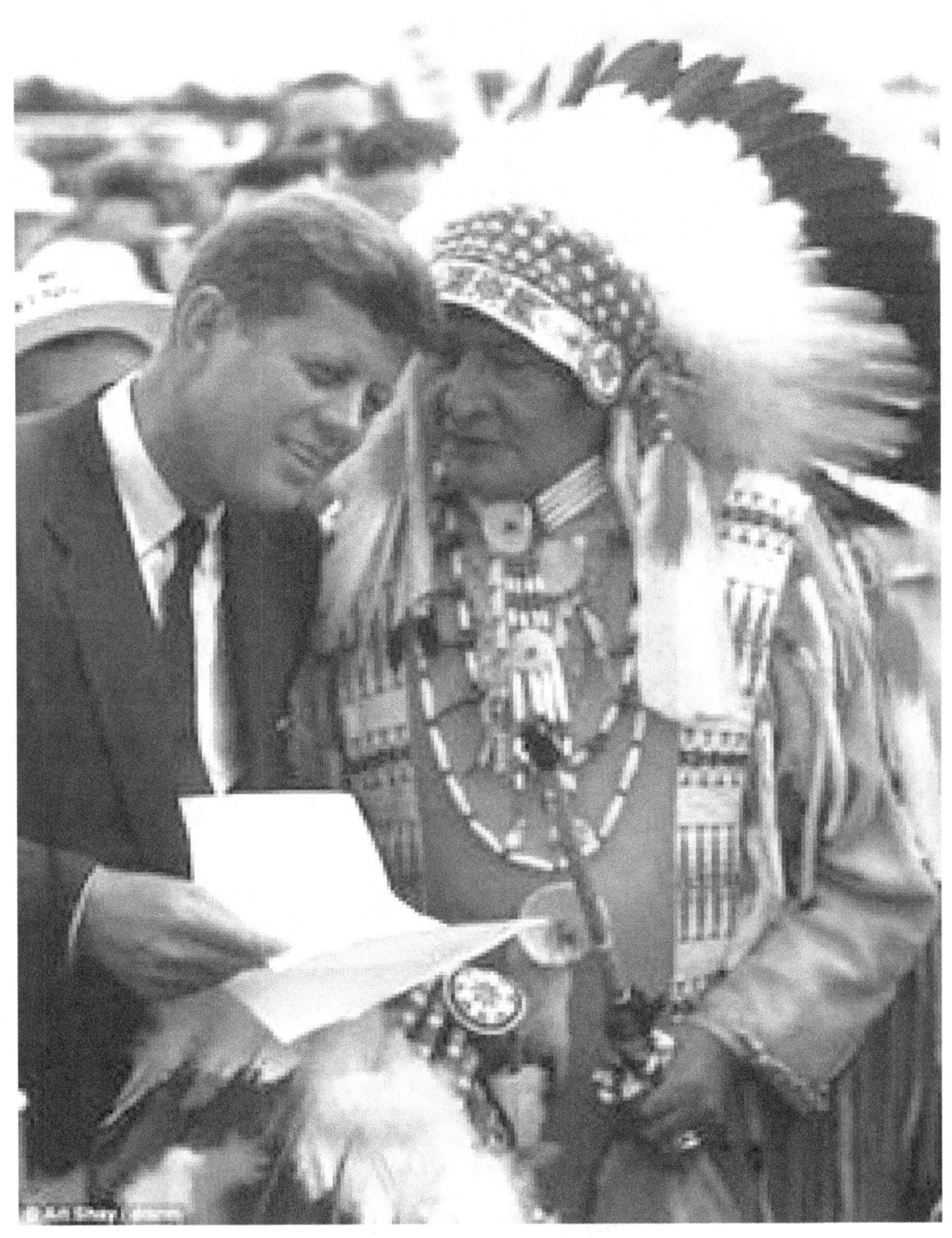

Who Knew?

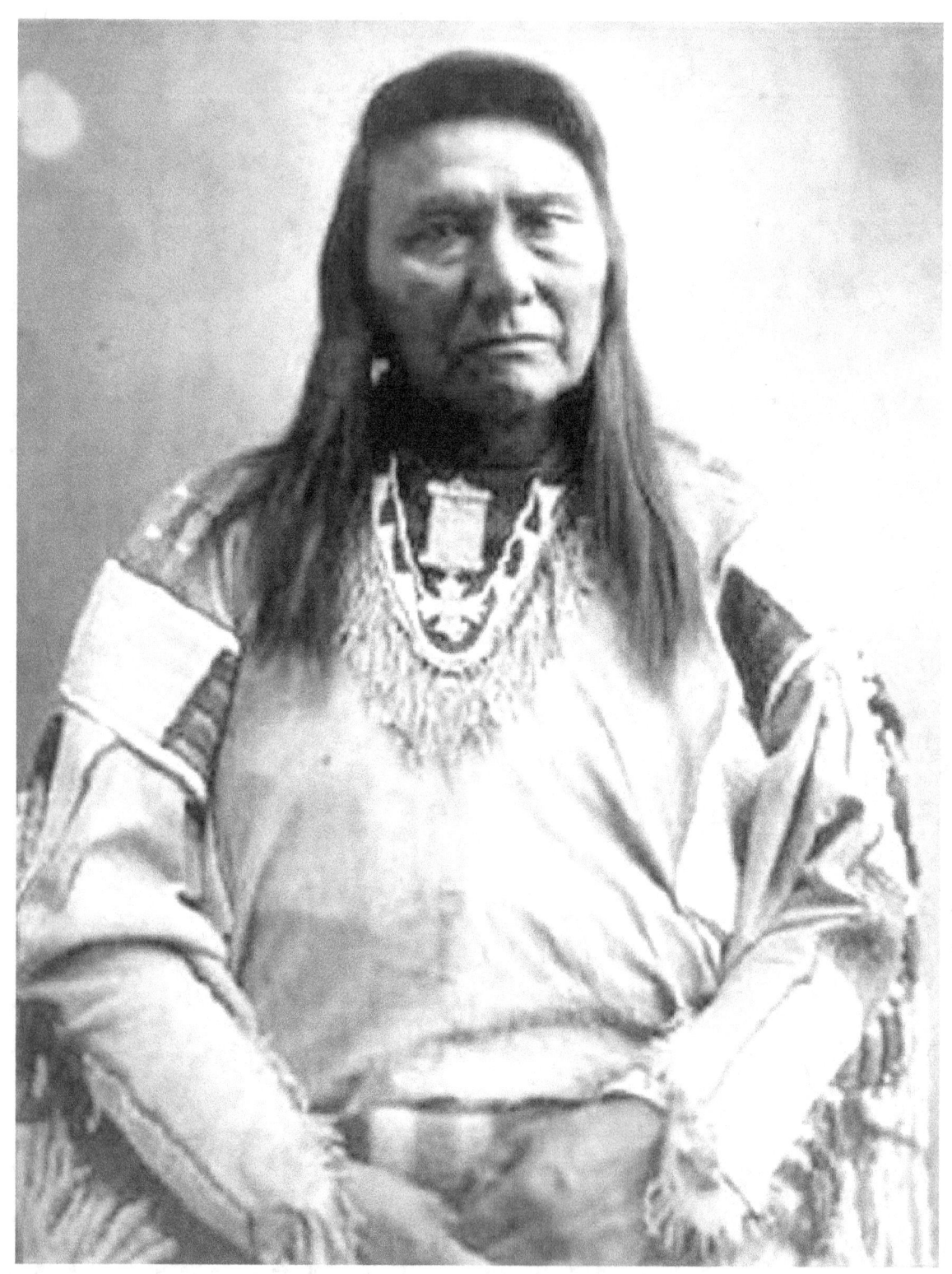

Chief Joseph, Nez Perce

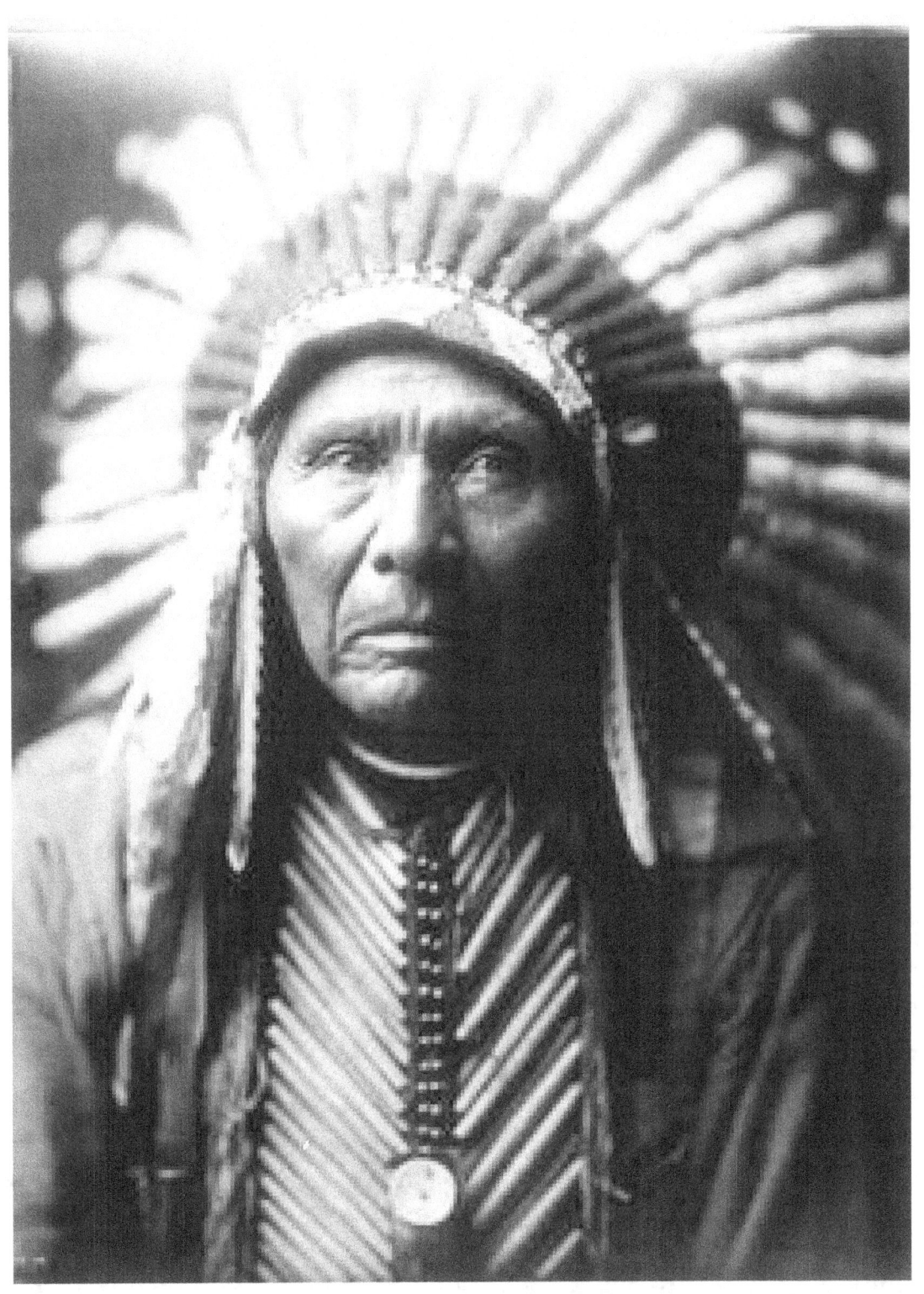

Three Horses, by Edward Curtis

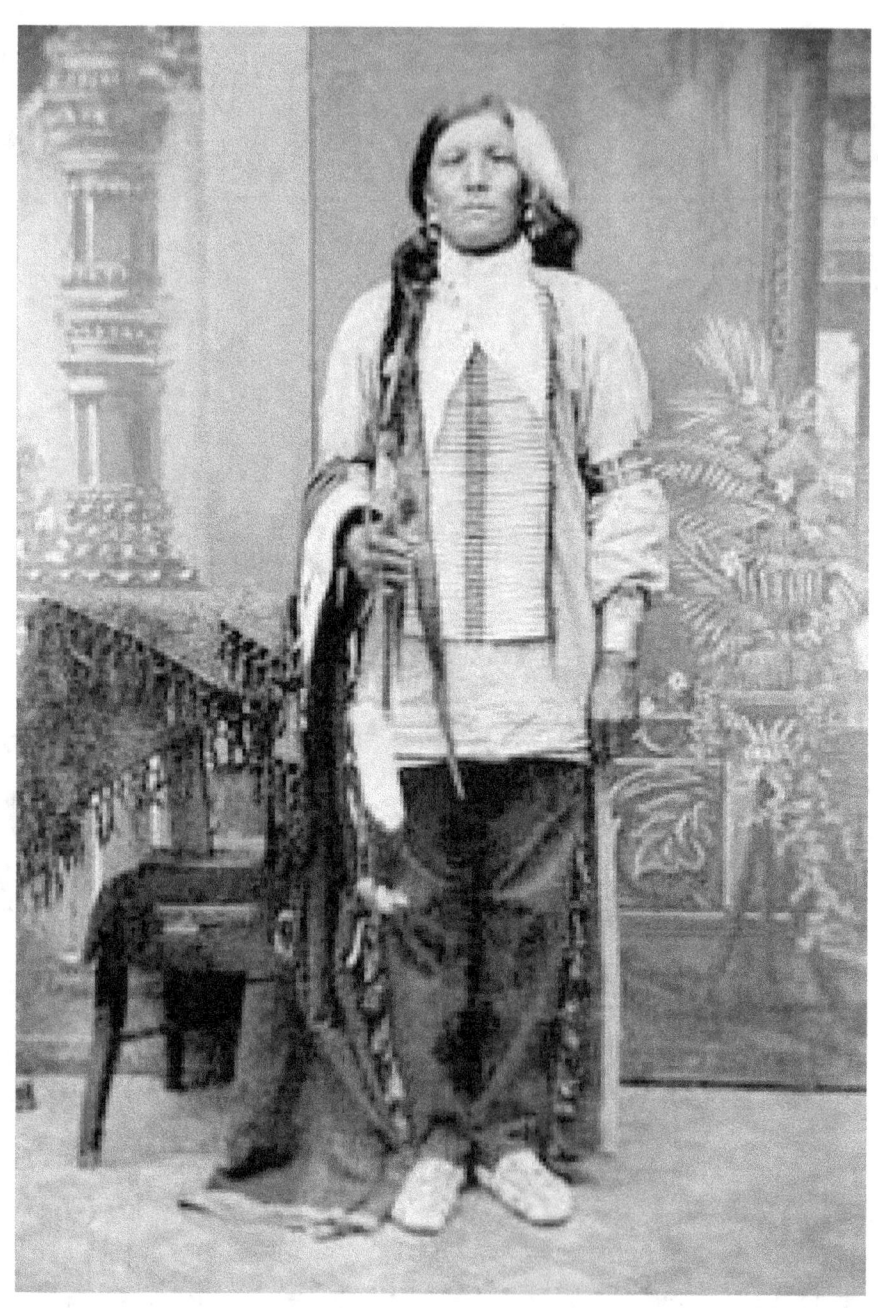

Ťhašúŋke Witkó, ("His-Horse-is-Crazy" - Crazy Horse), 1849-1877. "I see a time of Seven Generations when all the colors of mankind will gather under the Sacred Tree of Life and the whole Earth will become one circle again. In that day, there will be those among the Lakota who will carry knowledge and understanding of unity among all living things and the young white ones will come to those of my people and ask for this wisdom."

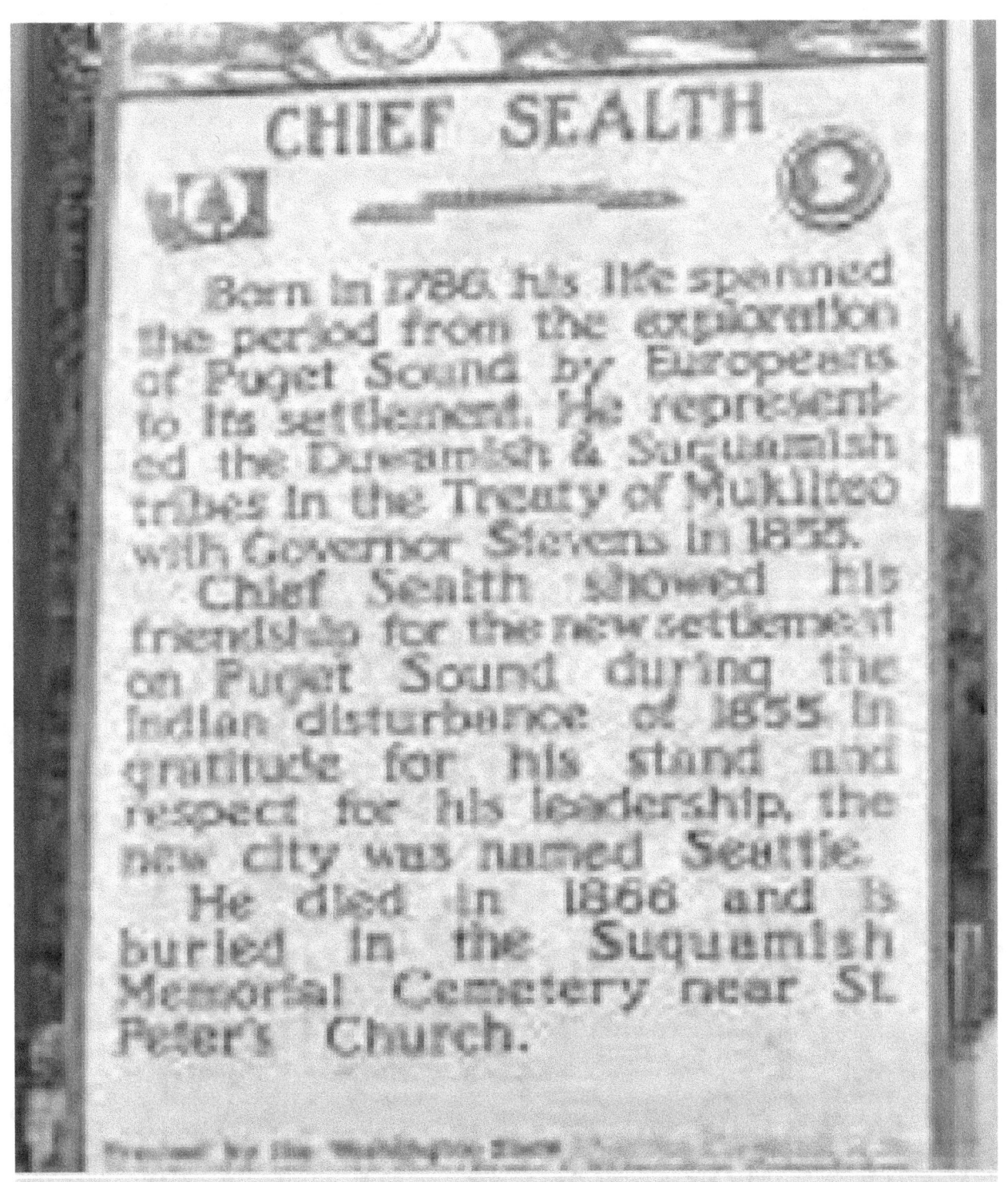

CHIEF SEALTH

Born in 1786, his life spanned the period from the exploration of Puget Sound by Europeans to its settlement. He represented the Duwamish & Suquamish tribes in the Treaty of Mukilteo with Governor Stevens in 1855.

Chief Sealth showed his friendship for the new settlement on Puget Sound during the Indian disturbance of 1855. In gratitude for his stand and respect for his leadership, the new city was named Seattle.

He died in 1866 and is buried in the Suquamish Memorial Cemetery near St. Peter's Church.

Erected by the Washington State ...

Chief Seattle's Monument

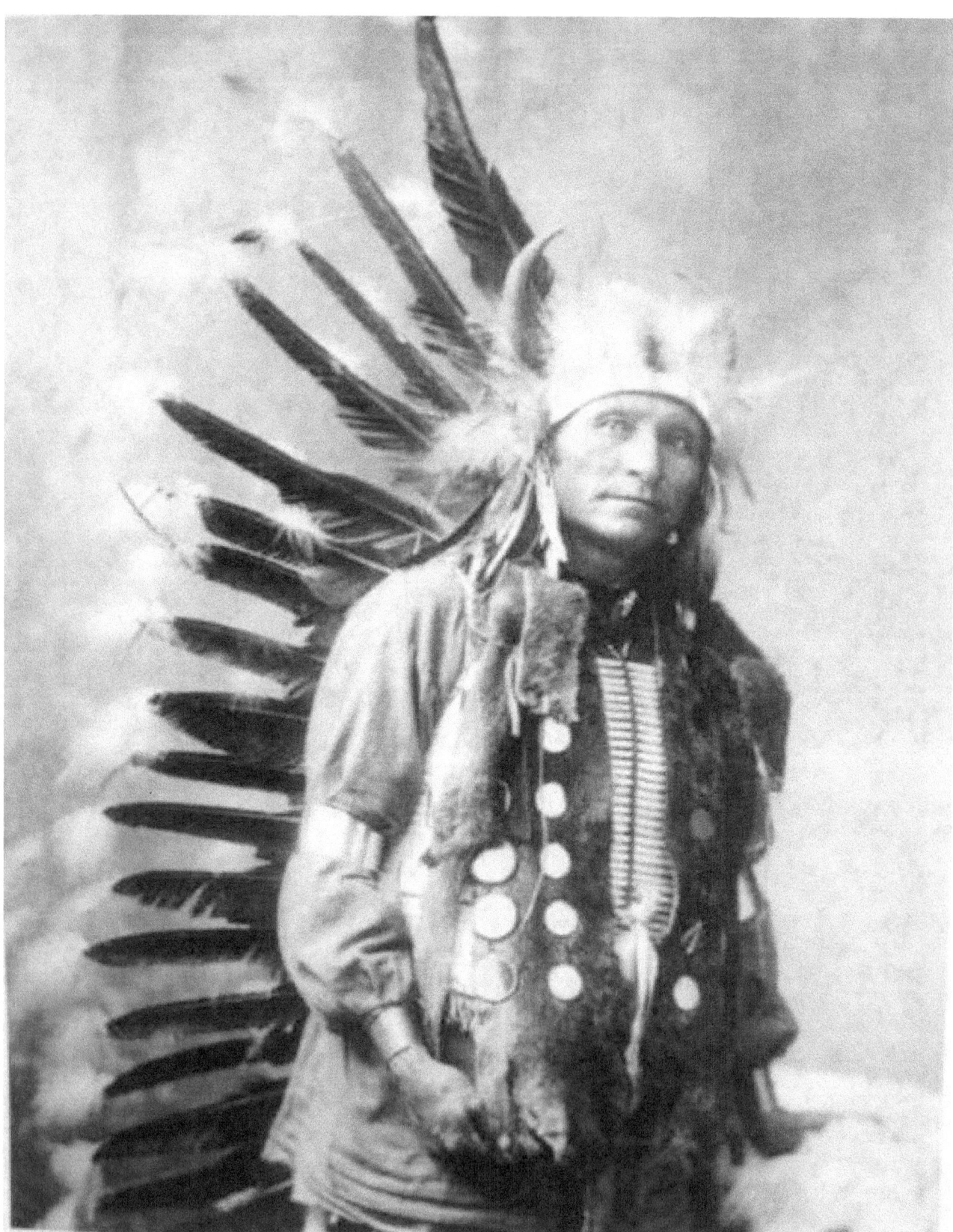

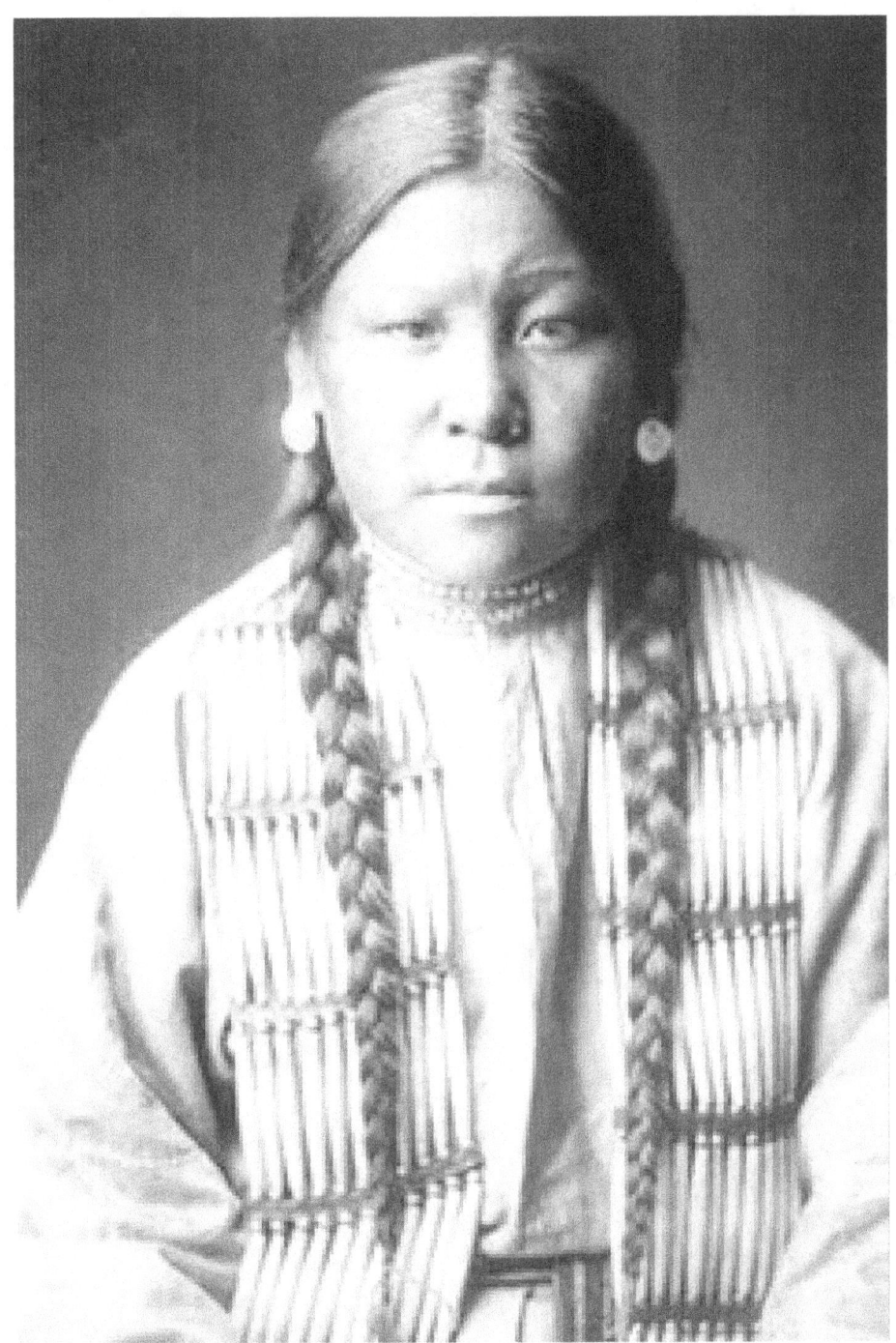

Buffalo Calf Road Woman (1850s-1878), was a Northern Cheyenne woman who saved her wounded warrior brother Chief Comes in Sight, in the Battle of Rosebud (as it was called by the US) in 1876. She fought next to her husband in the Battle of the Little Bighorn that same year. In 2005 Northern Cheyenne storytellers broke more than 100 years of silence about the battle, and they credited her with striking the blow that knocked General George Armstrong Custer off his horse before he died.

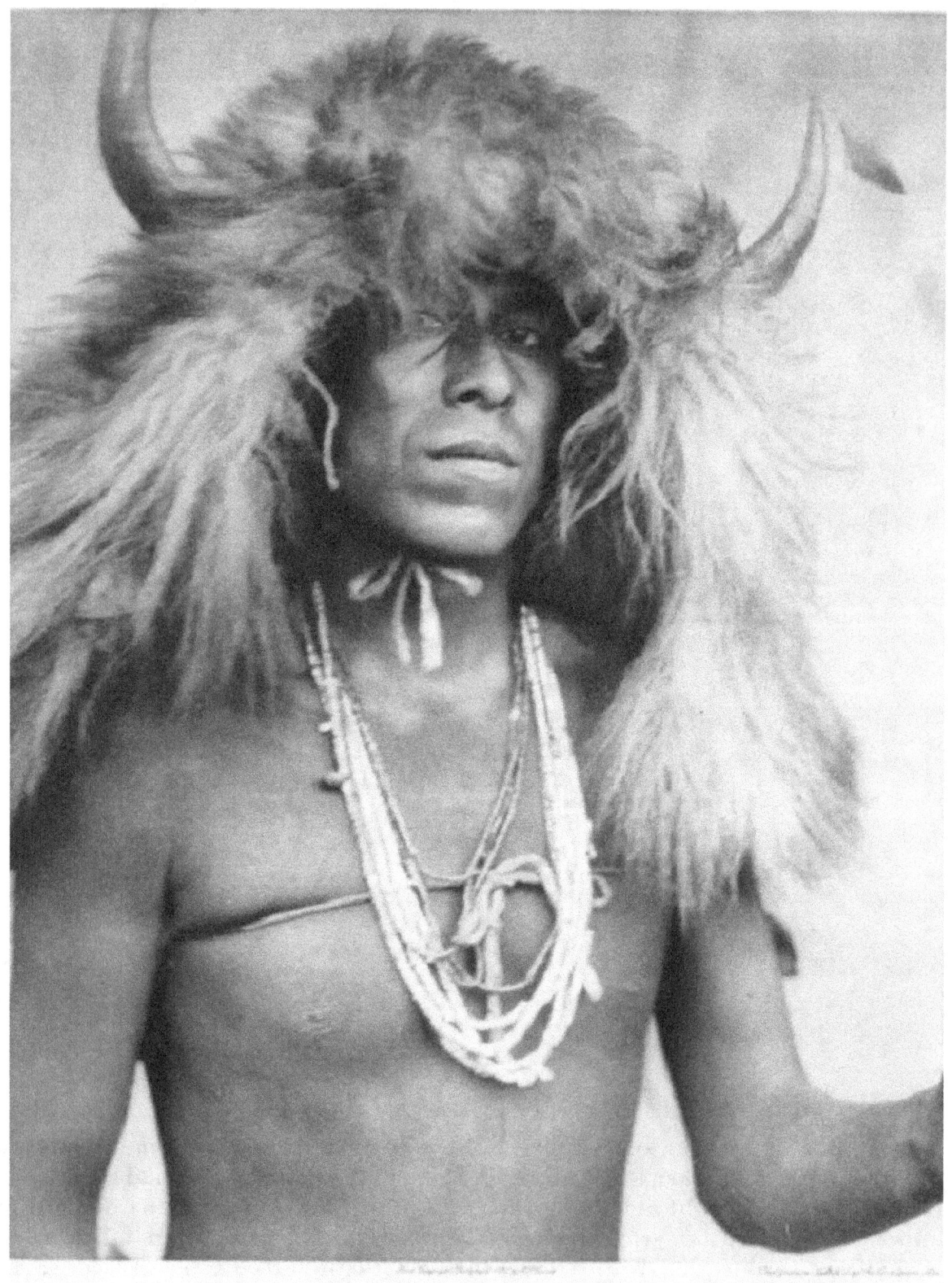

SIA BUFFALO MASK

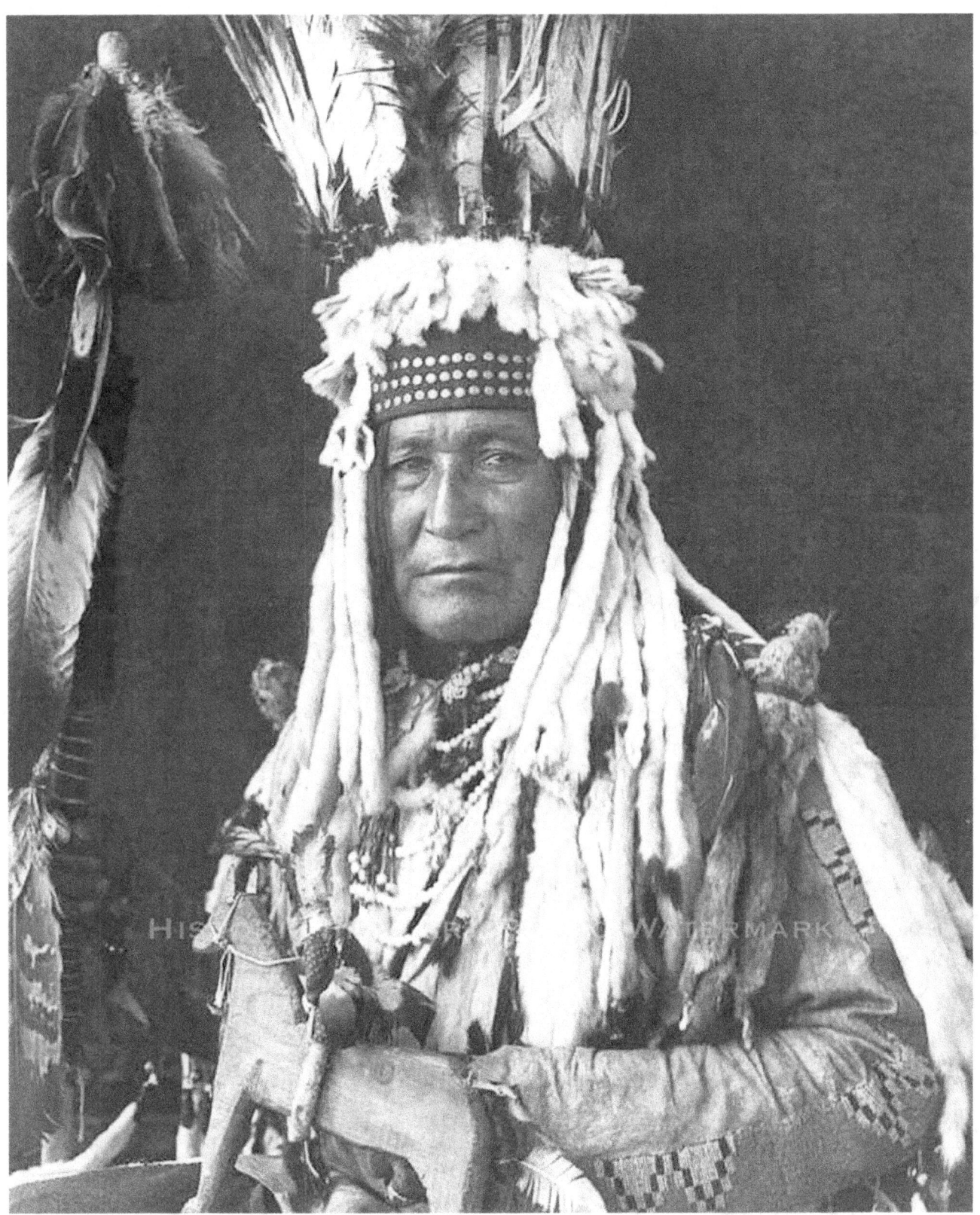

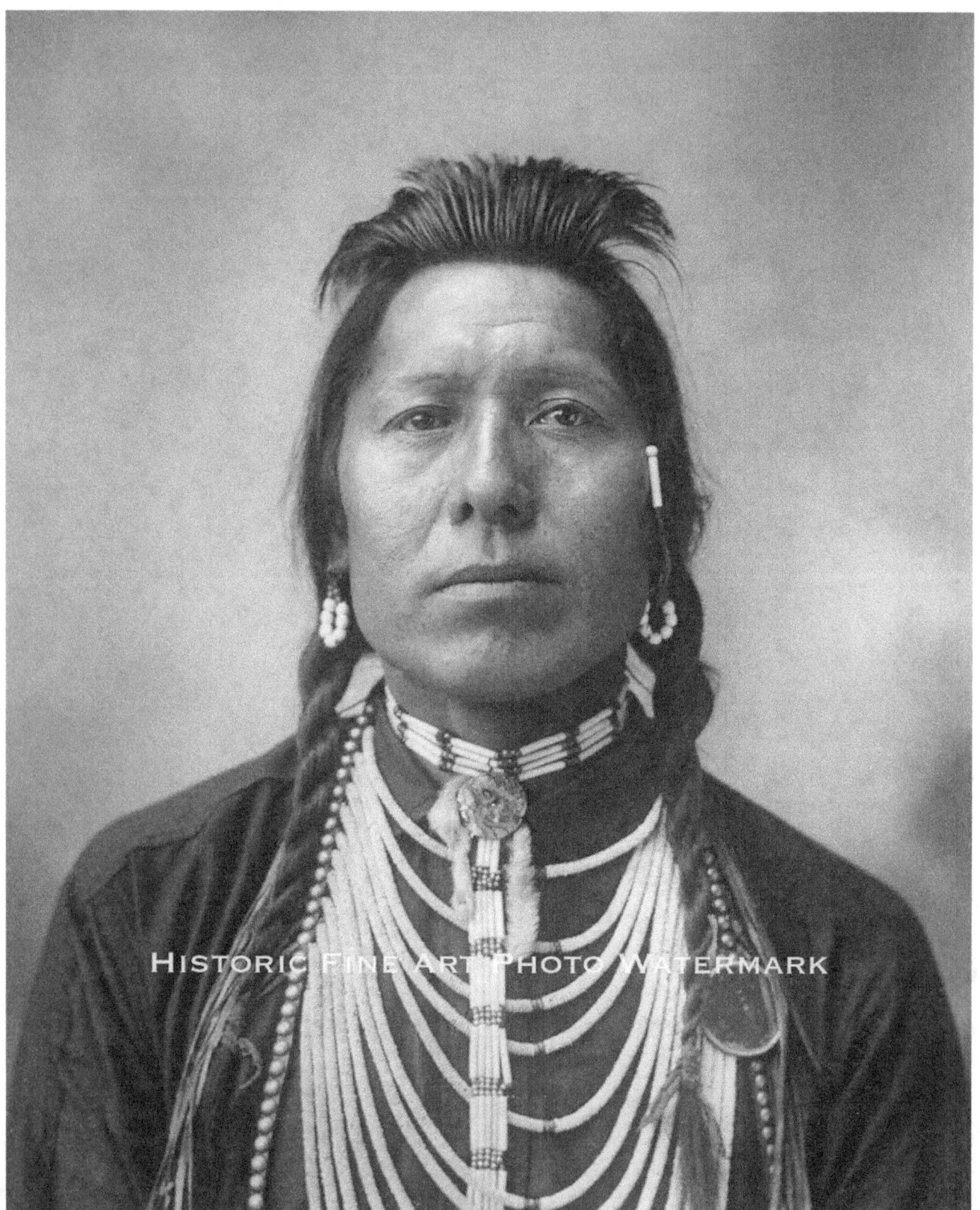

liv

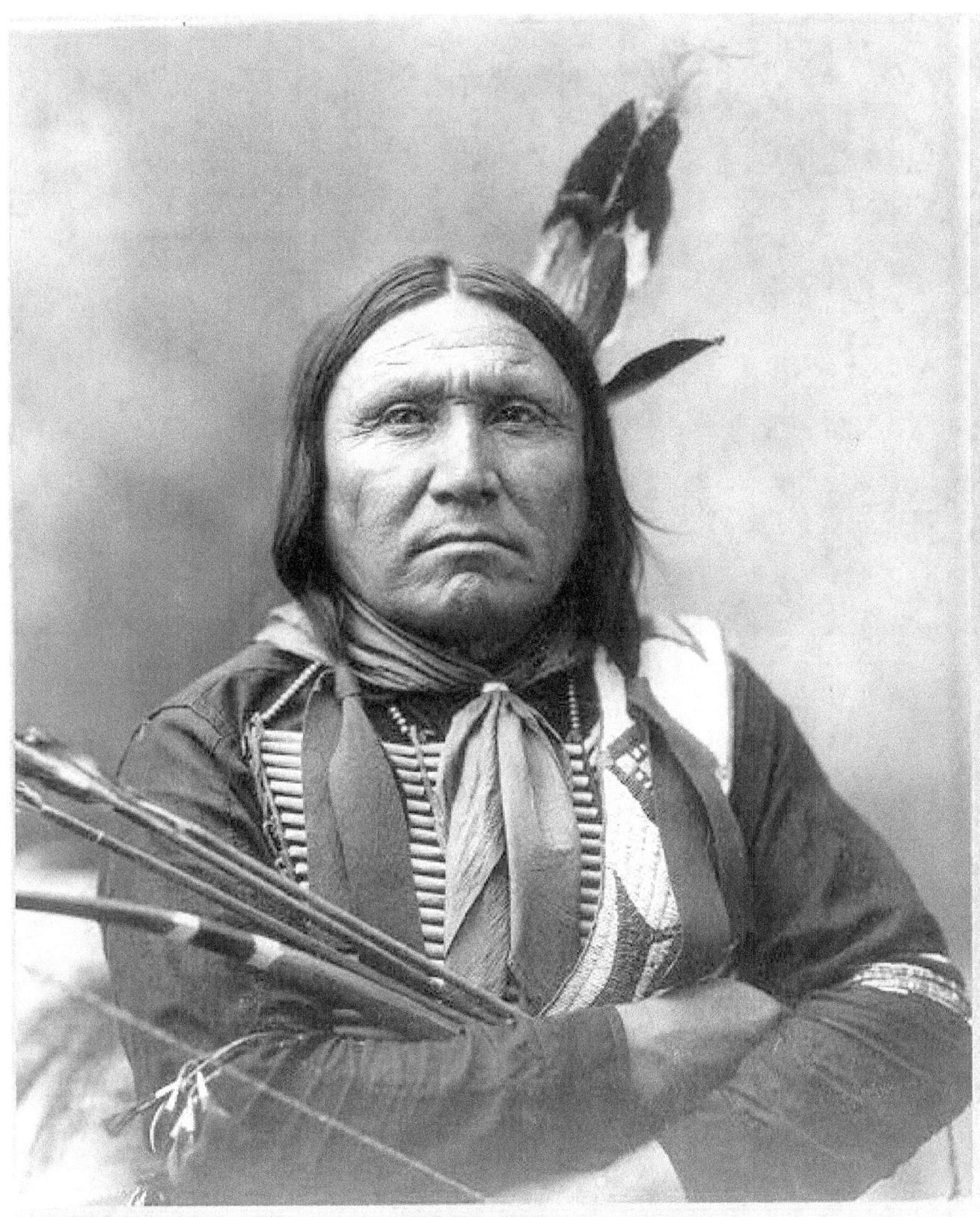

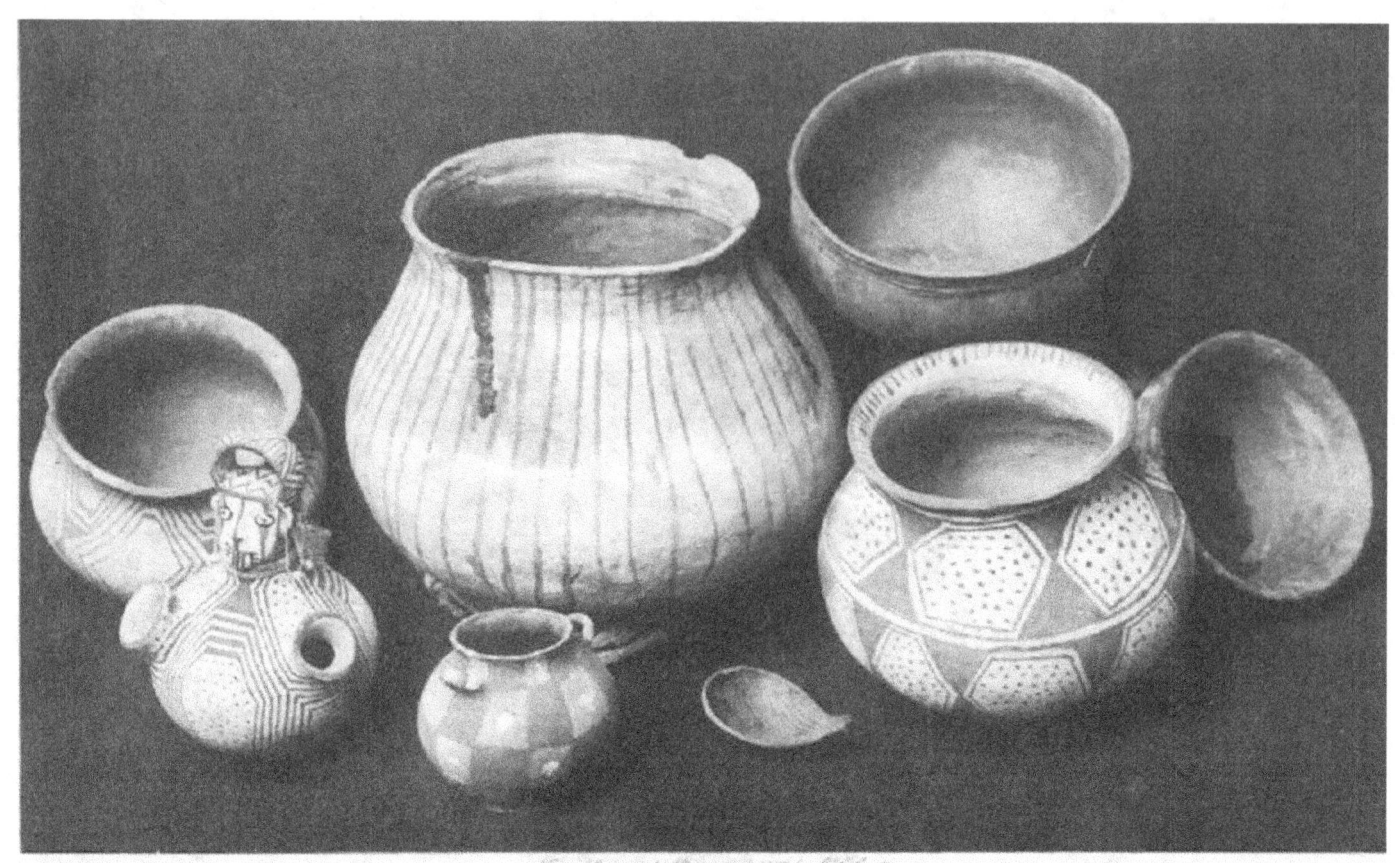

MOHAVE STILL LIFE

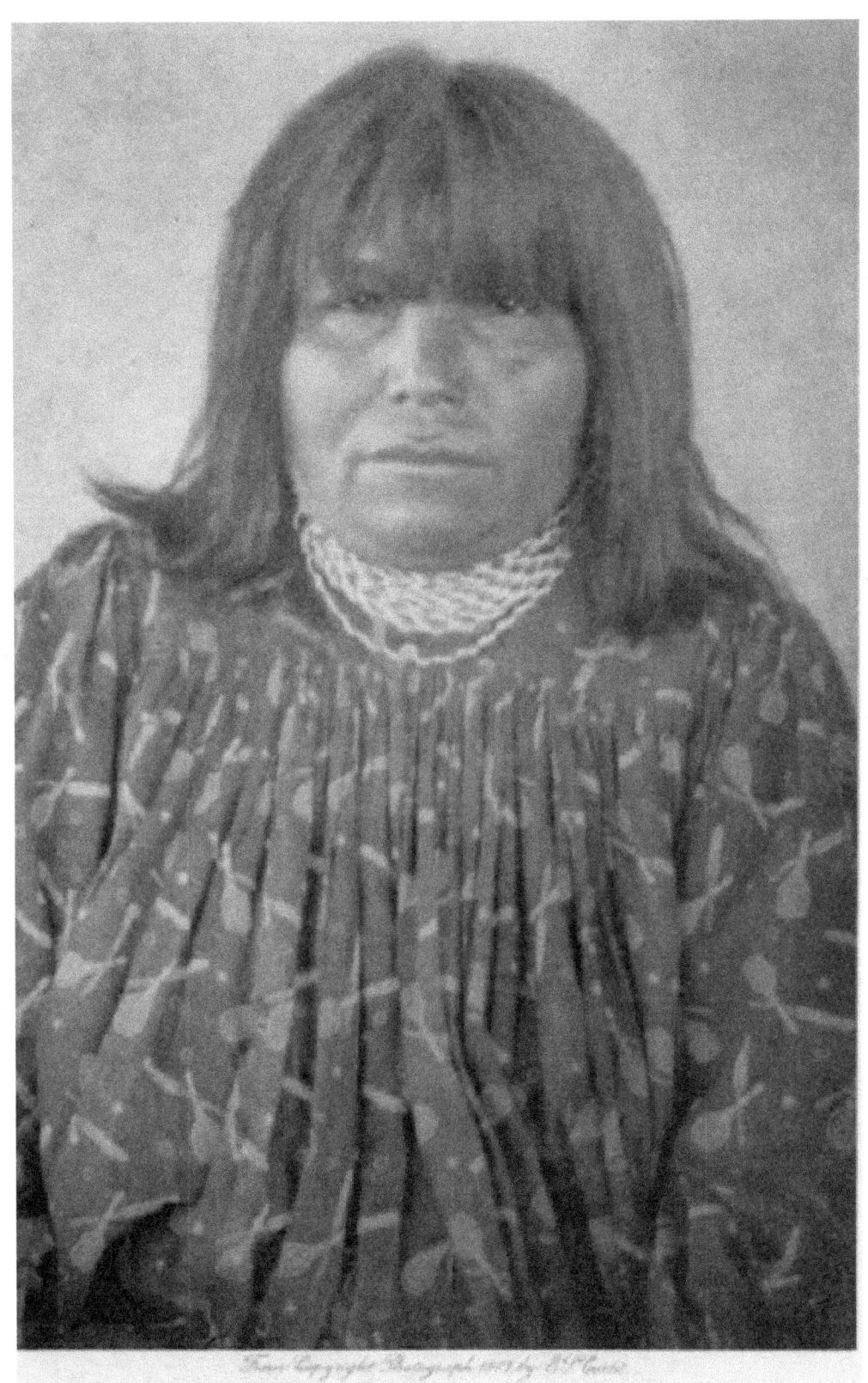

From Copyright Photograph 1903 by E. S. Curtis

APACHE MOHAVE WOMAN

lvii

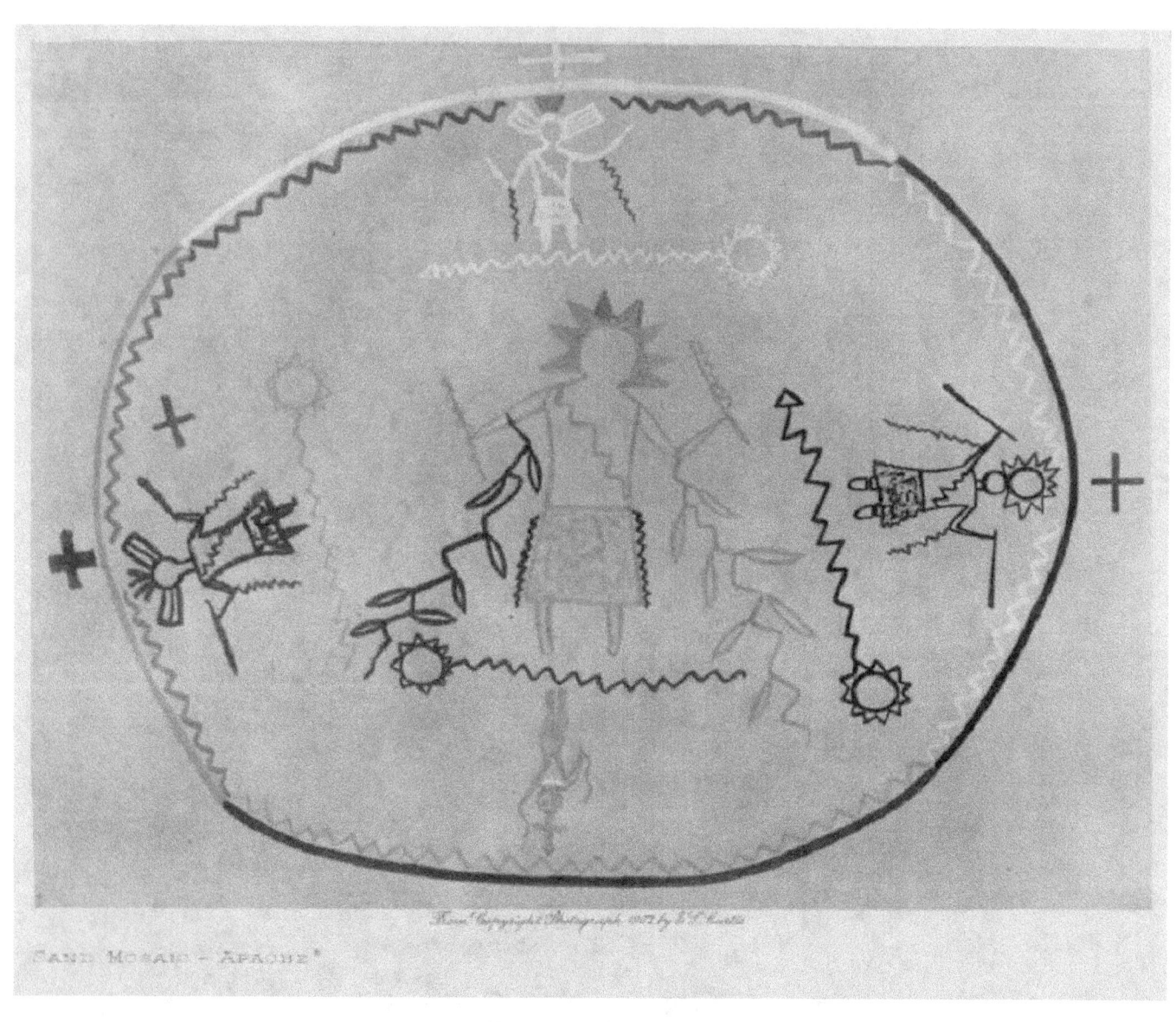

A Sand Mosaic – Apache

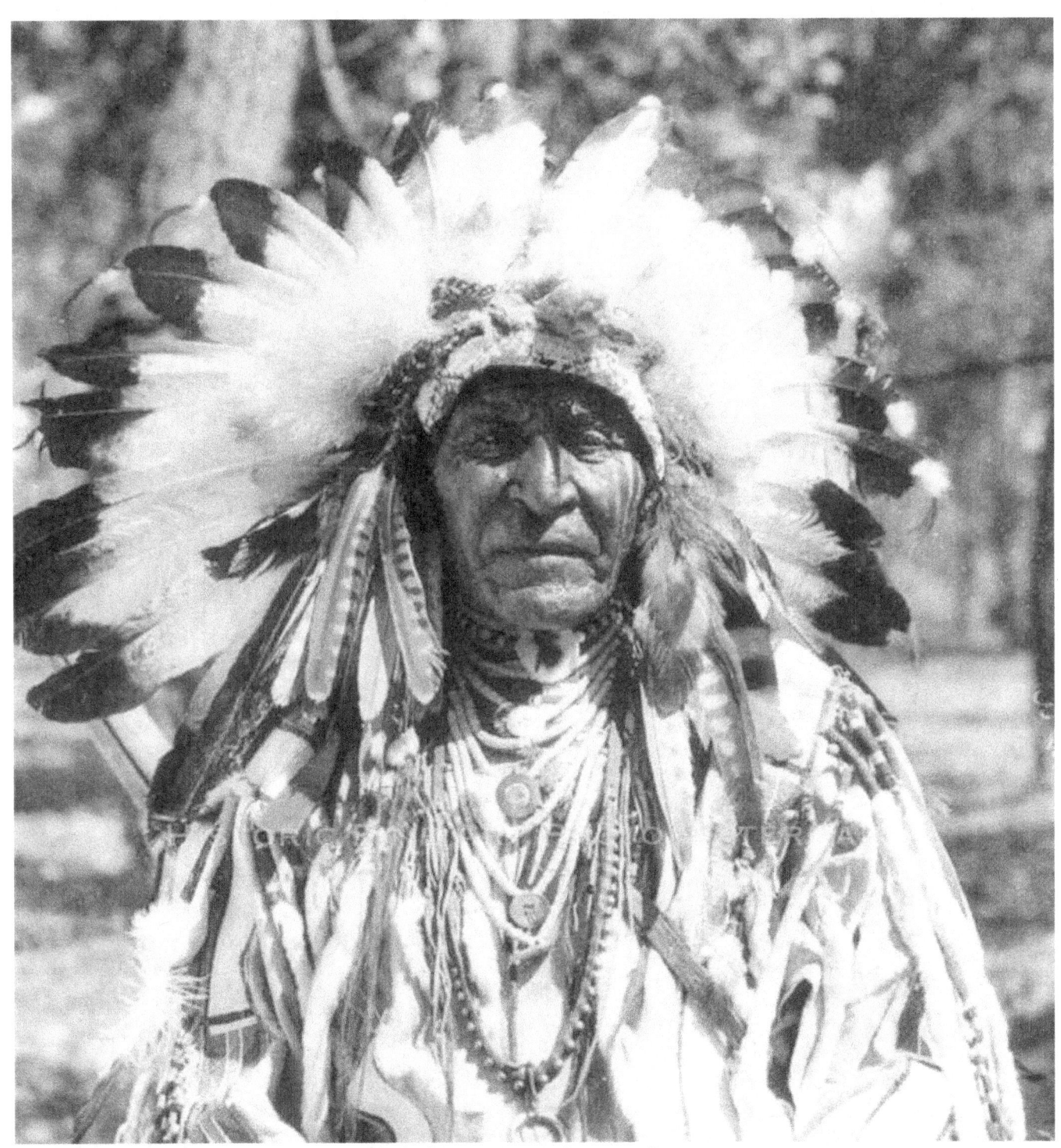

Chief Two Leggings - Crow

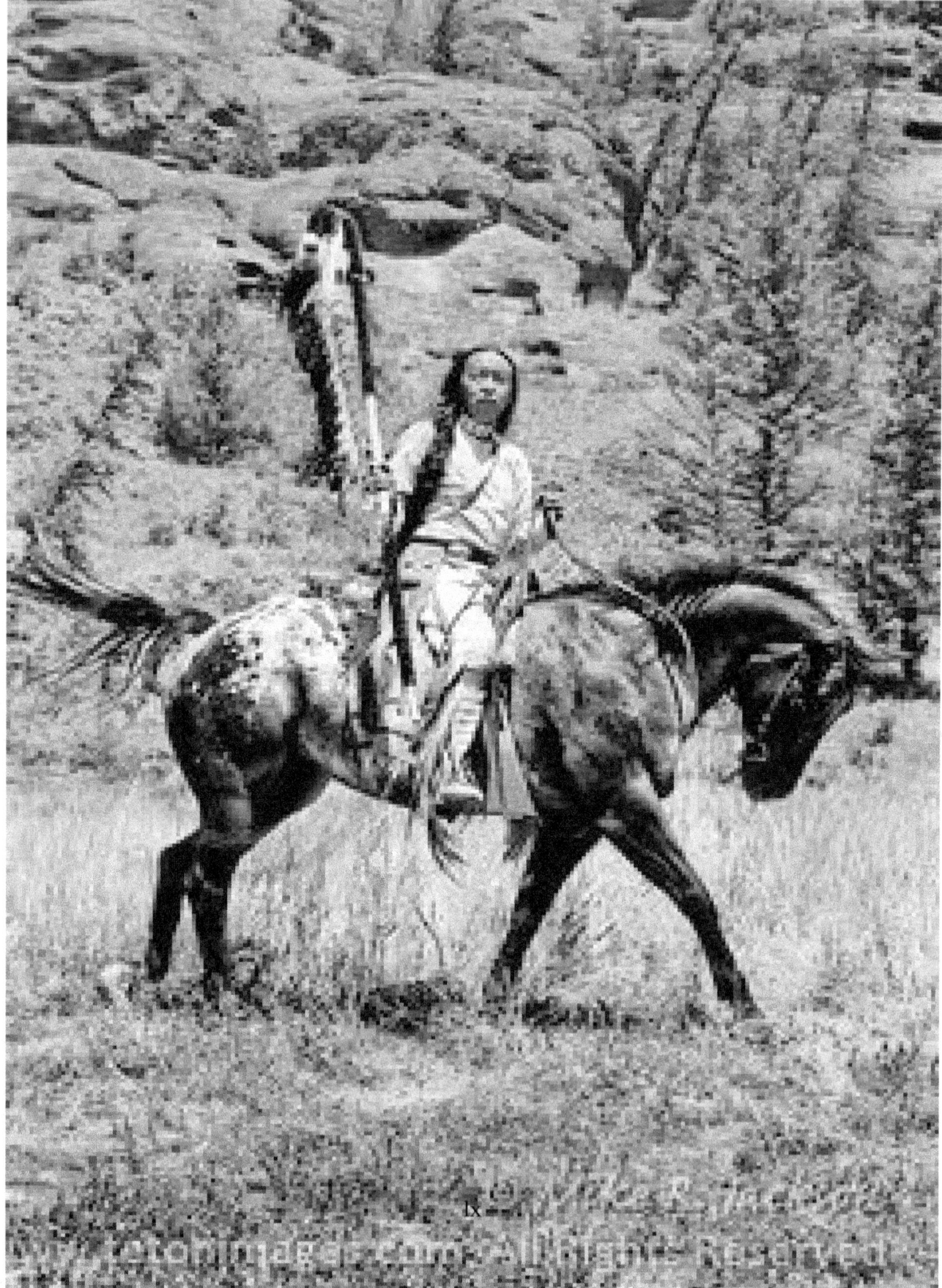

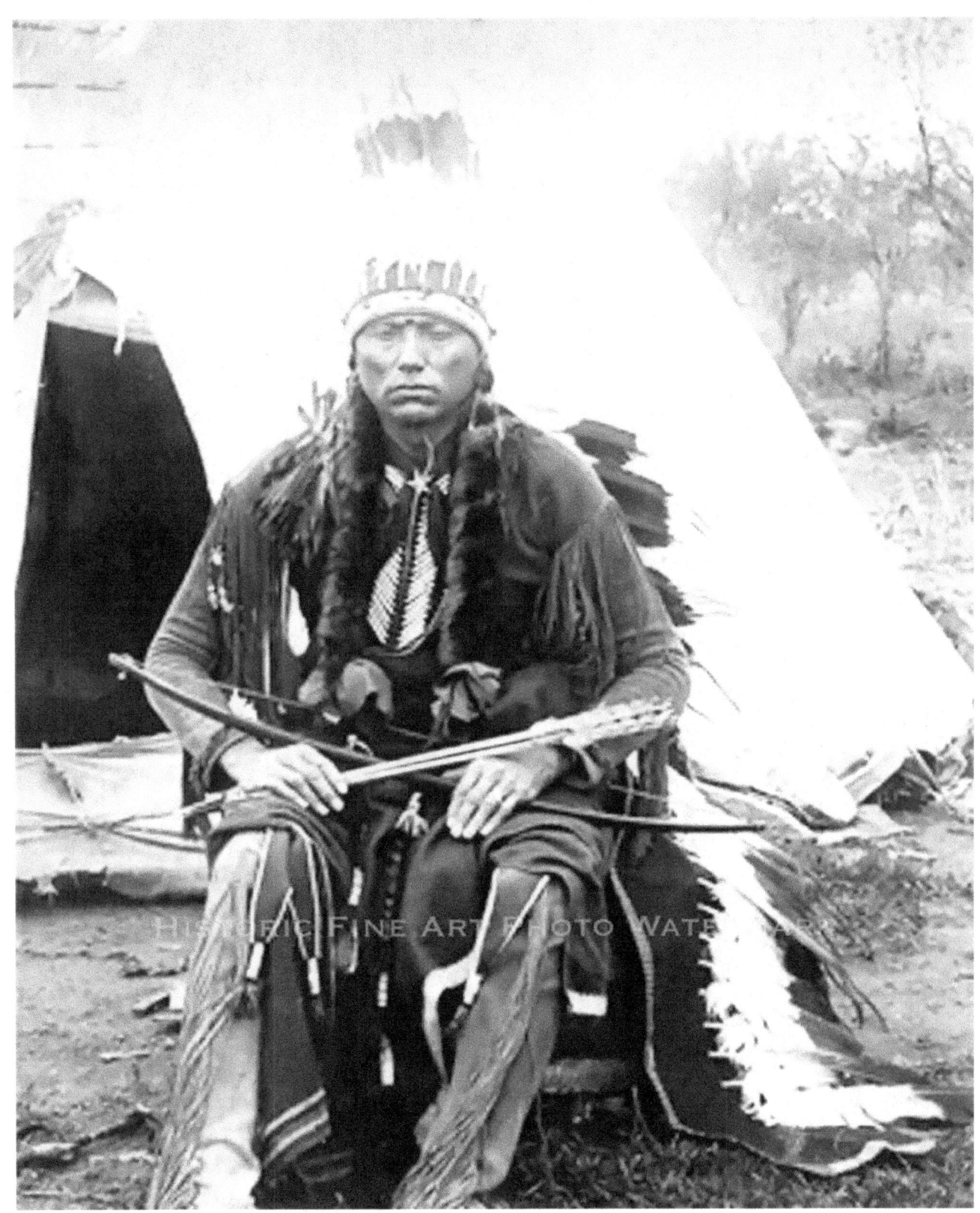

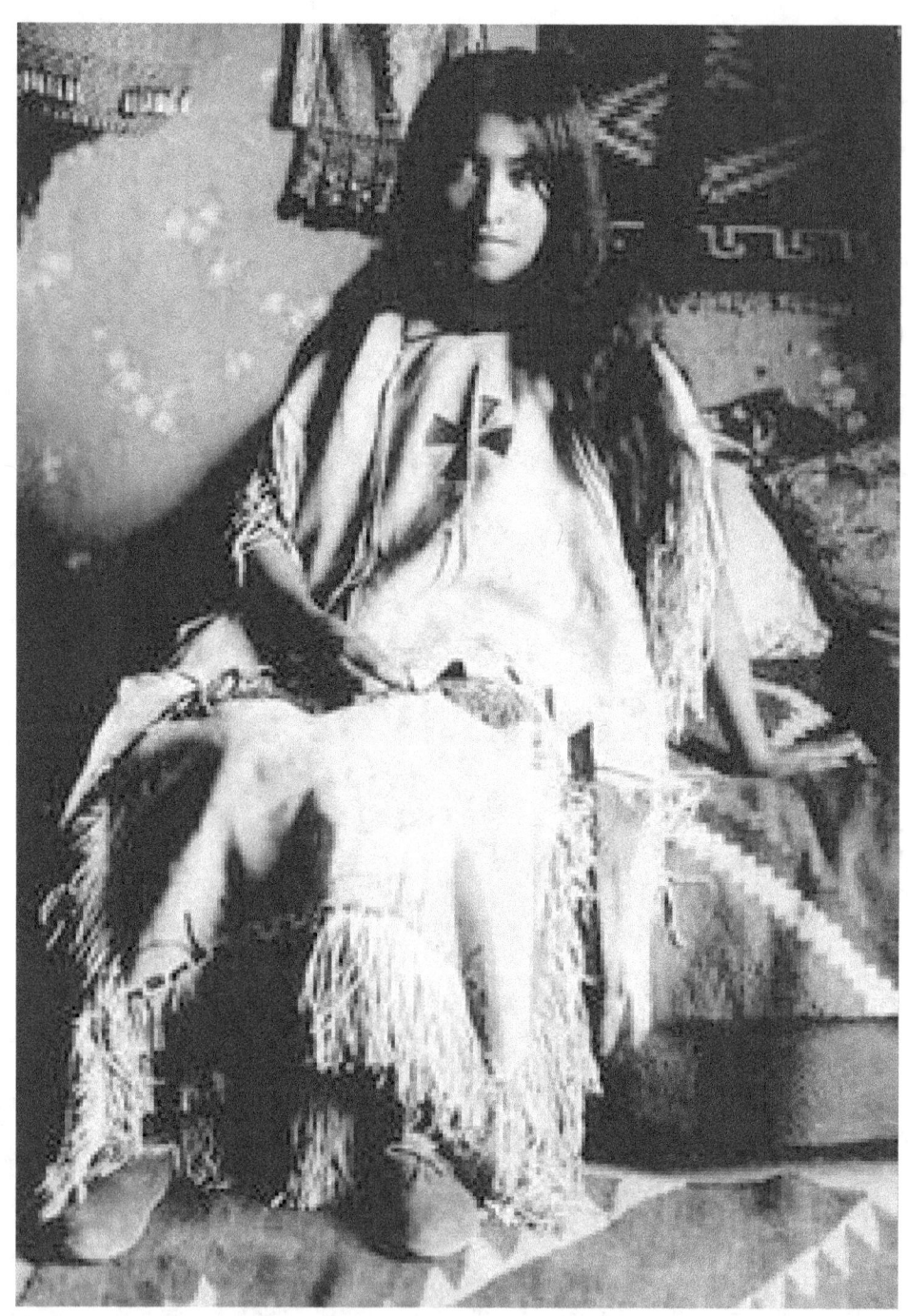

Beautiful daughter of Geronimo c.1900. - Lena Geronimo was born in 1886 in Fort Marion, St. Augustine, FL, while her father was a prisoner there. The medical staff gave her the name Marion, after the fort, but she took the name Lenna upon returning to the Southwest. Lenna Geronimo, the daughter of Geronimo and wife Ih-tedda, a Mescalero Apache, was the full sister of Robert Geronimo, Geronimo's only living son. Lenna was Bedonkohe- Mescalero.

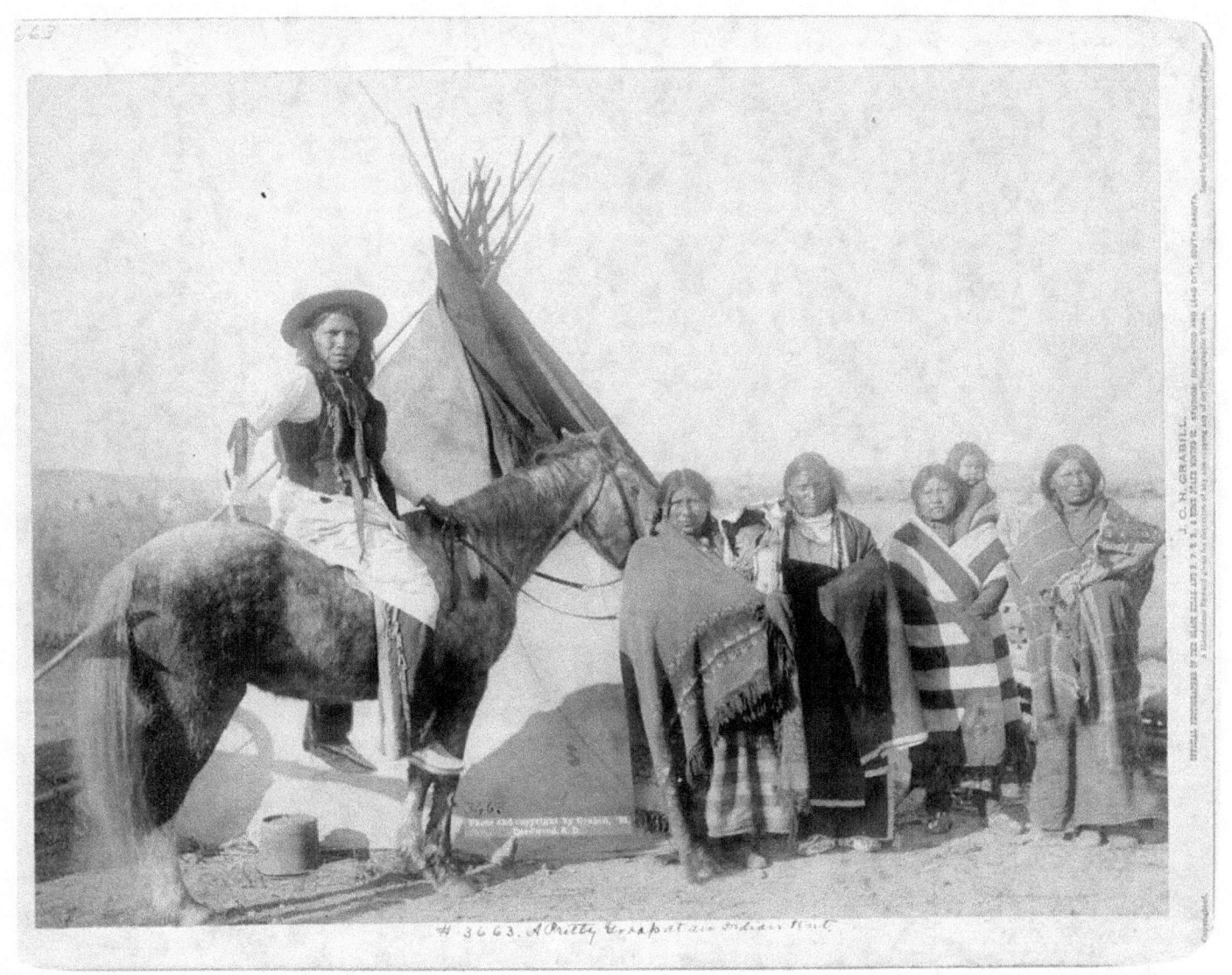

Pretty Group at a NativeTent. Taken near Pine Ridge by John C. H. Grabill, 1891.
blackhillsknowledgenetwork.org

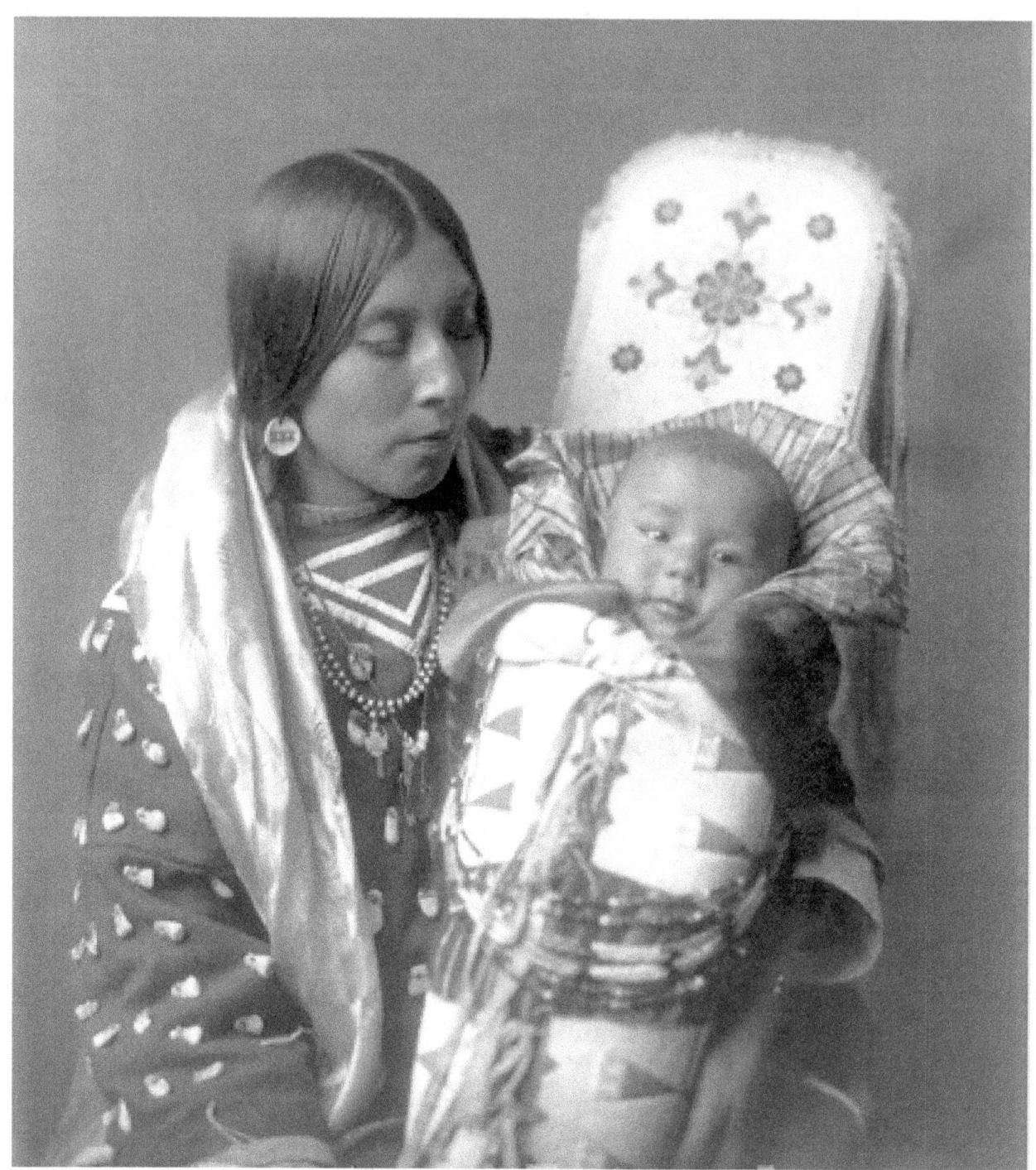

A Hopi Woman with her Papoose

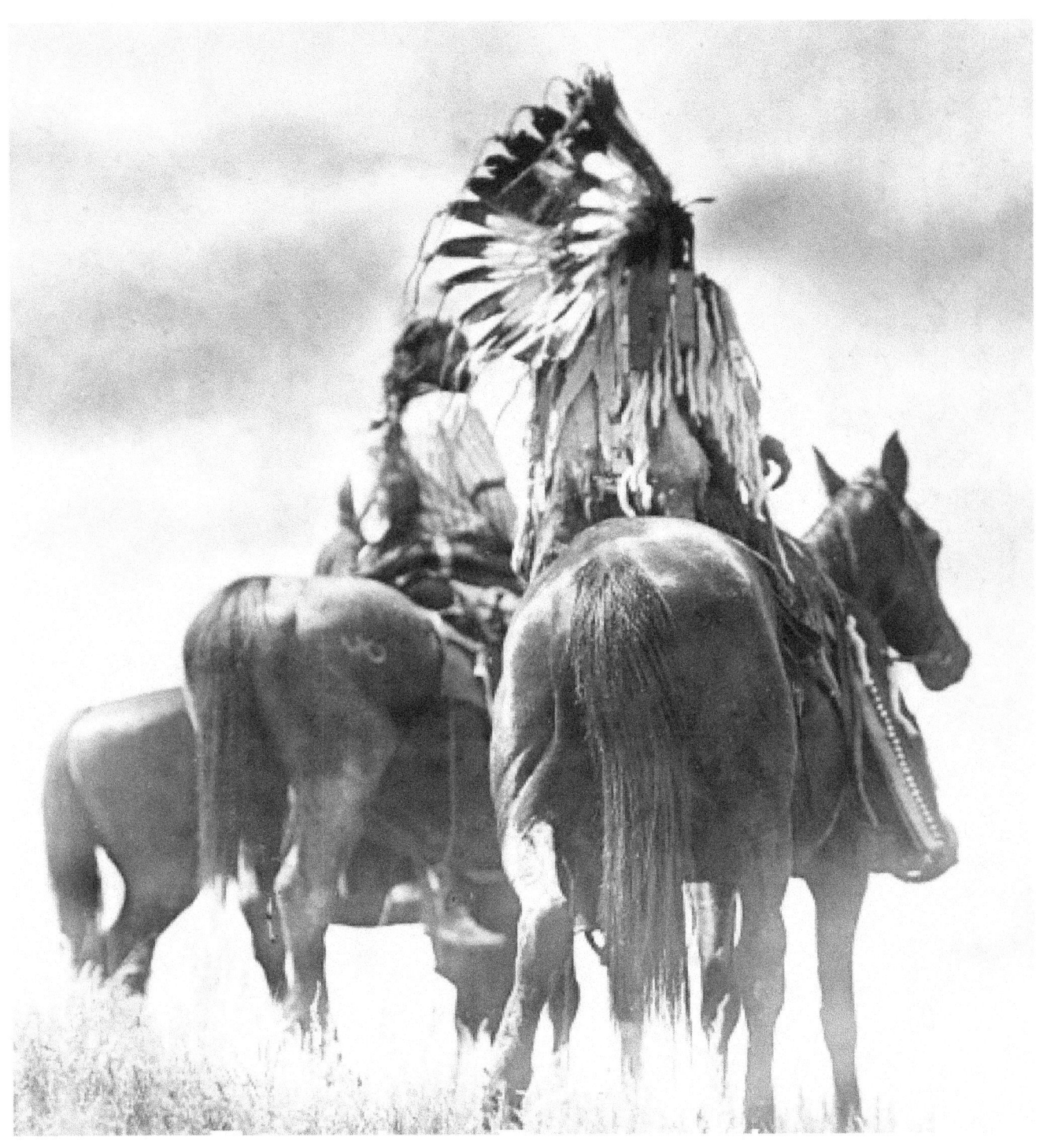

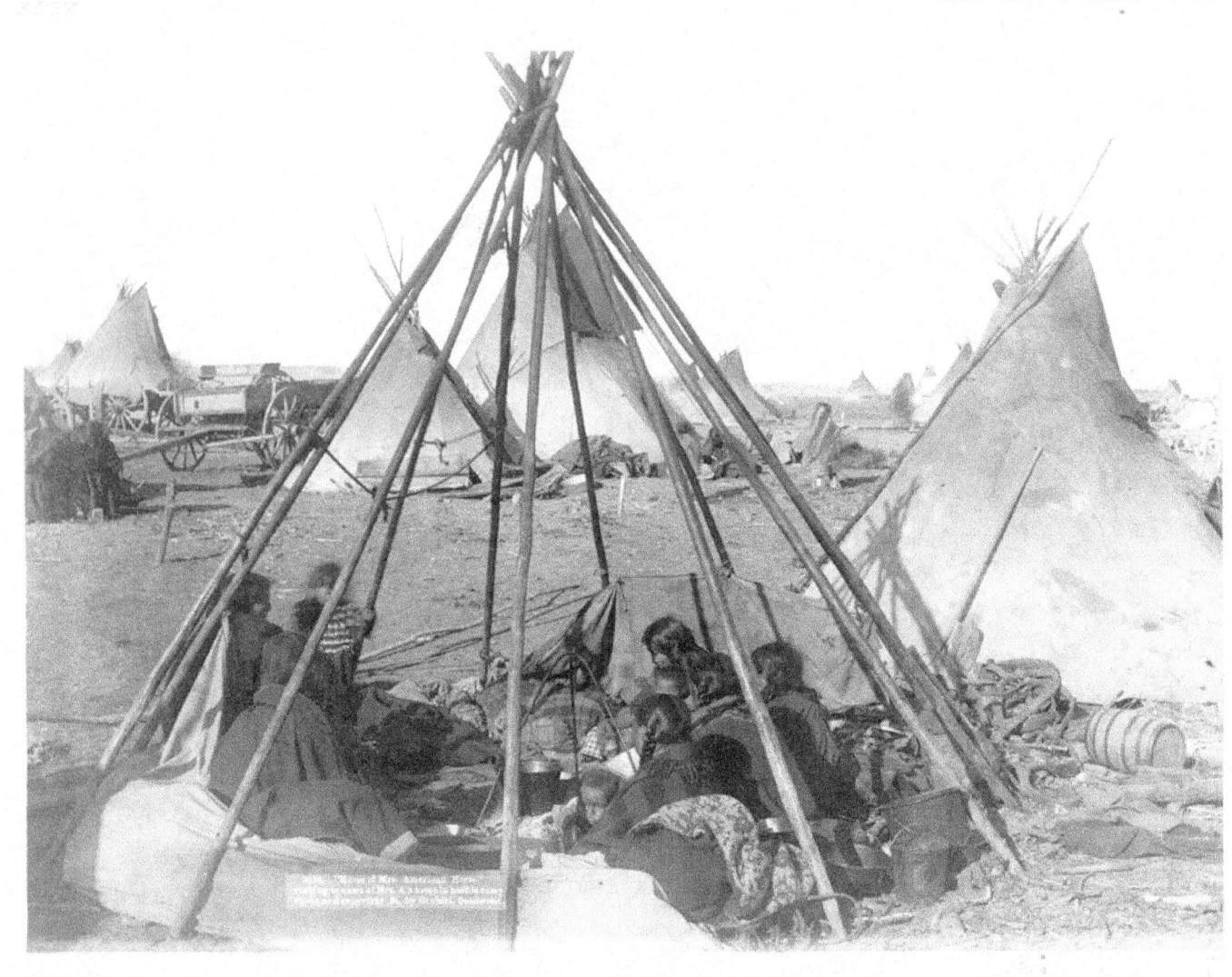

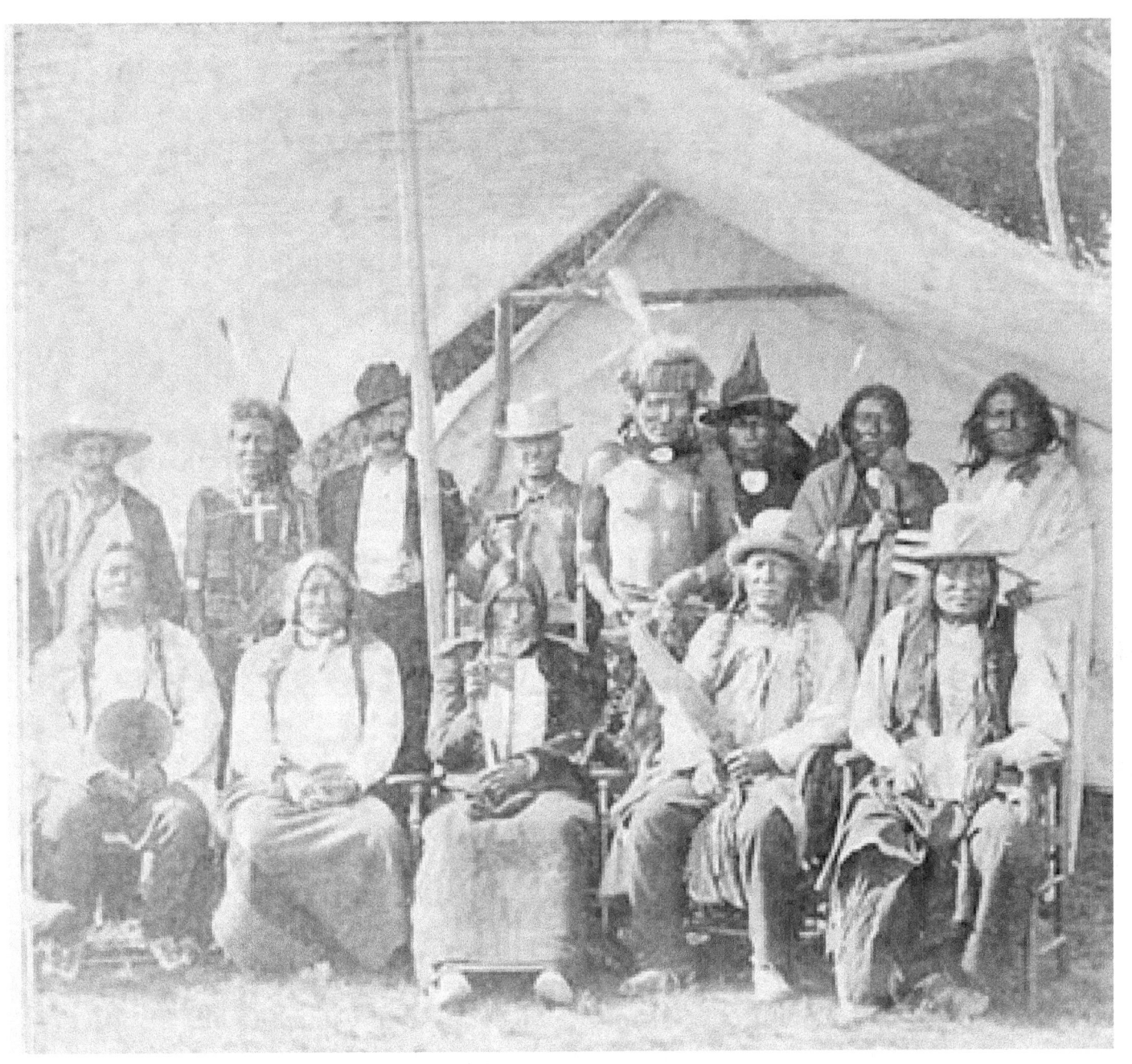

I'm sure this is Spotted Eagle second from the right of the back row

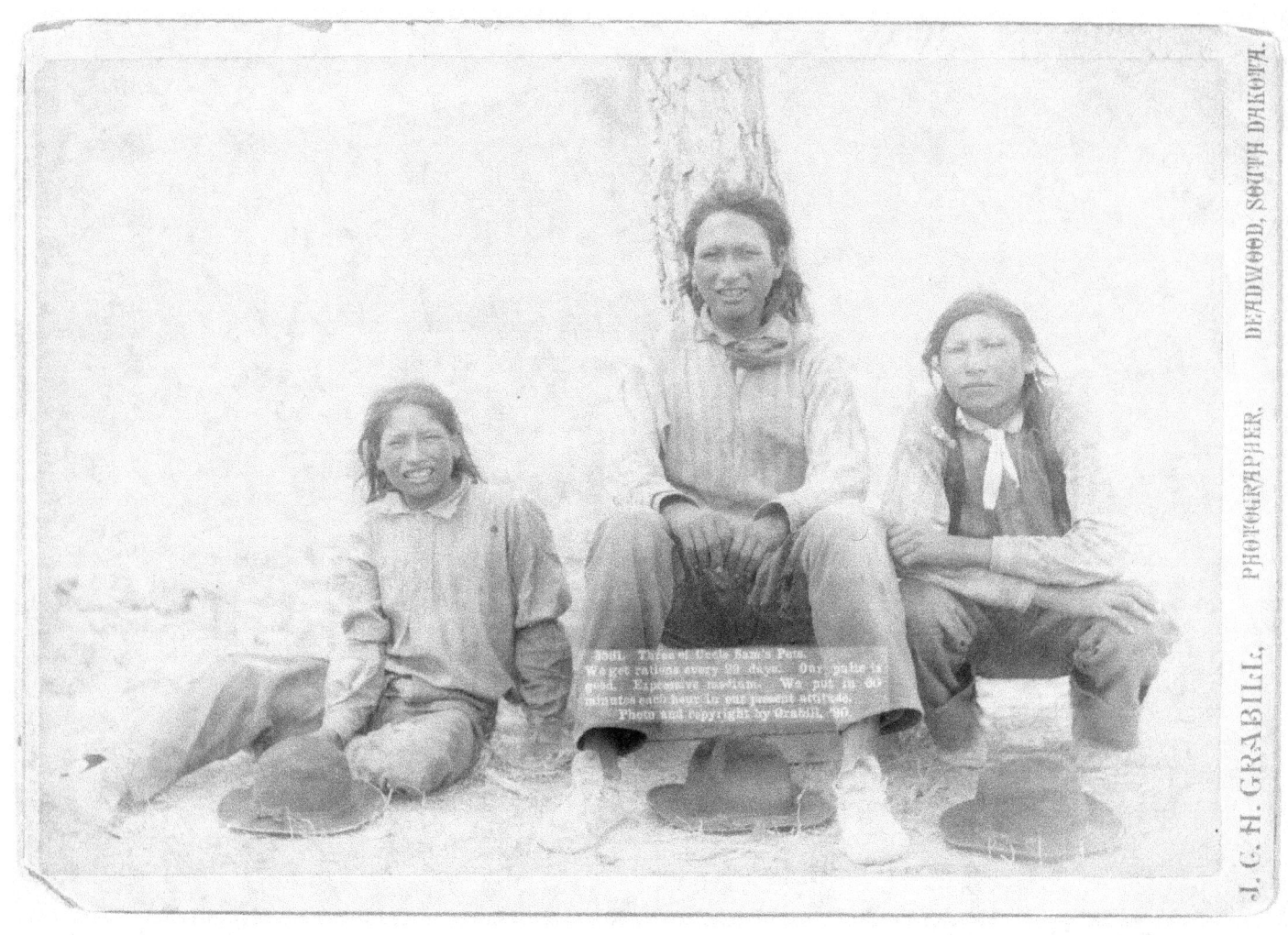

Lakota Teenagers, by John C. H. Grabill. The caption says, "Three of Uncle Sam's Pets. (!) We get rations every 29 days. Our pulse is good. Expressive medium. We put in 60 minutes each hour in our present attitude." 1890.
northwesthistory.blogspot.com

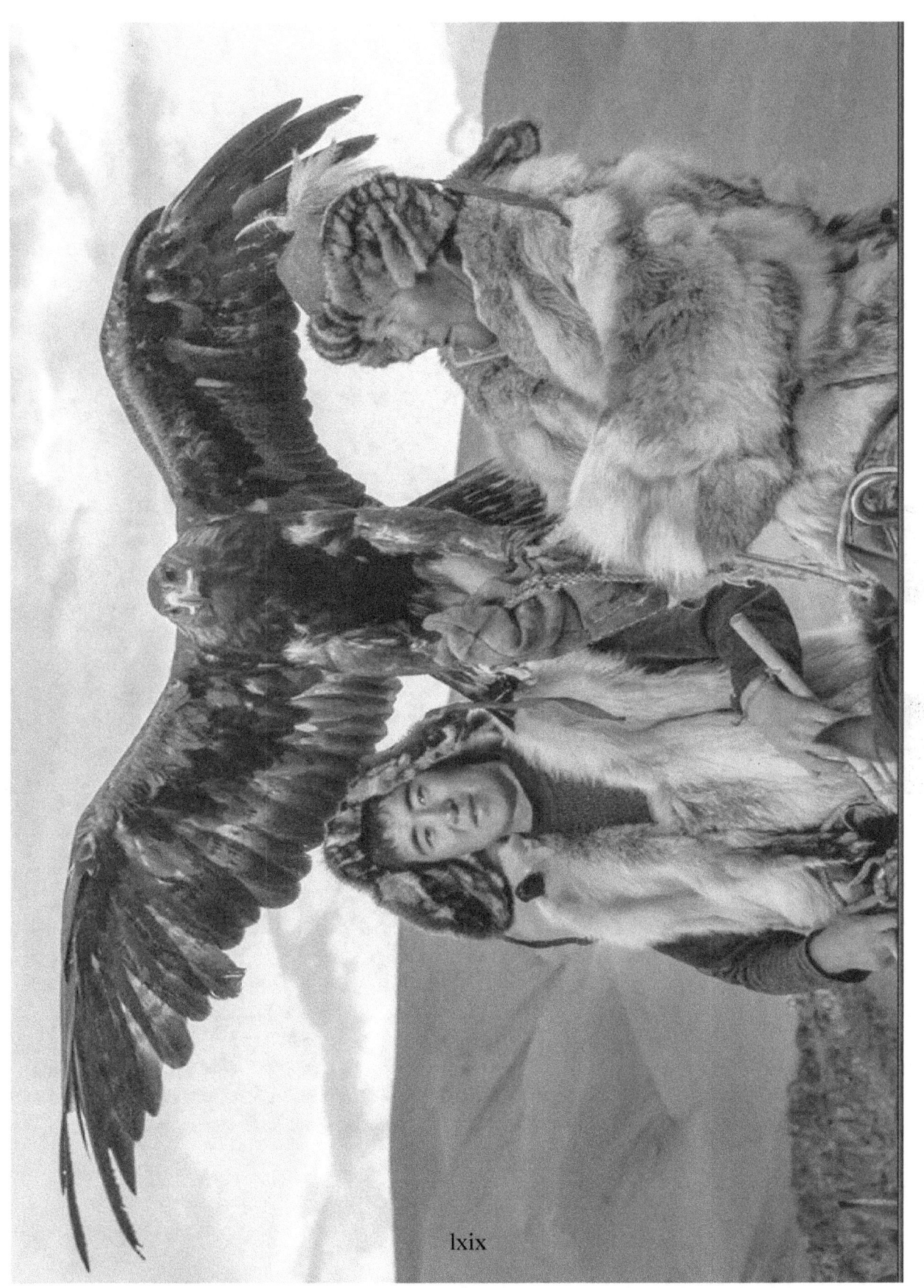

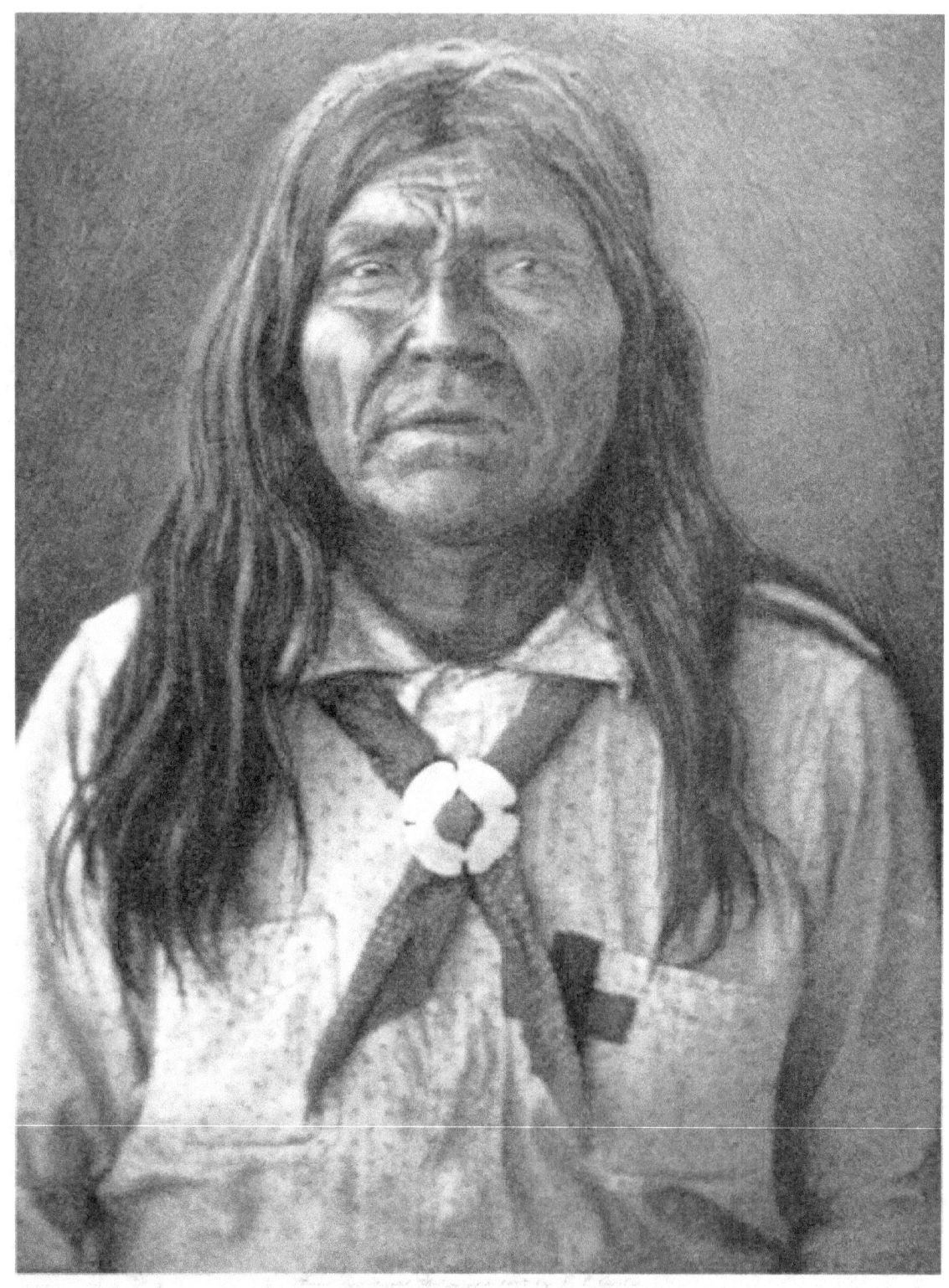

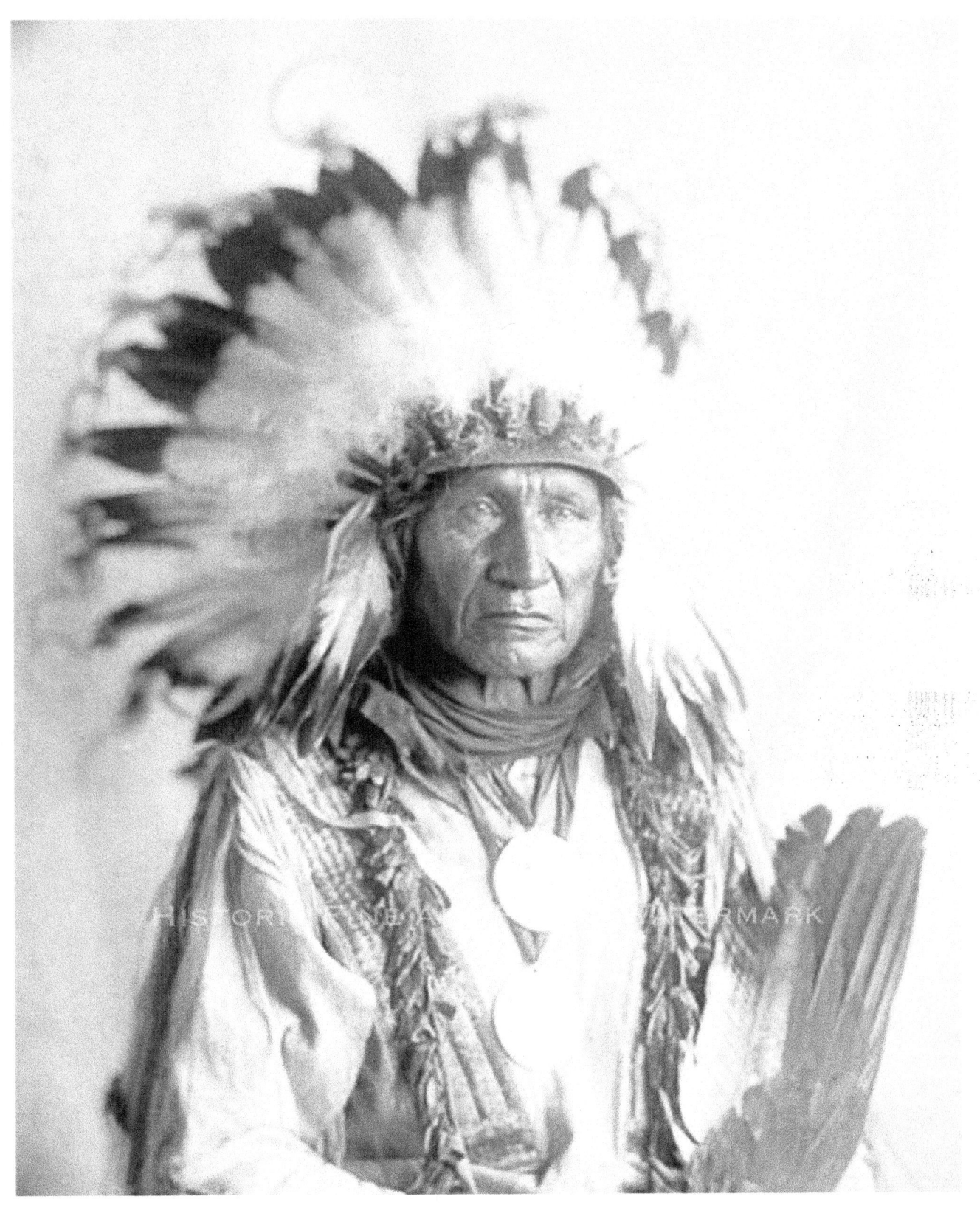

lxxi

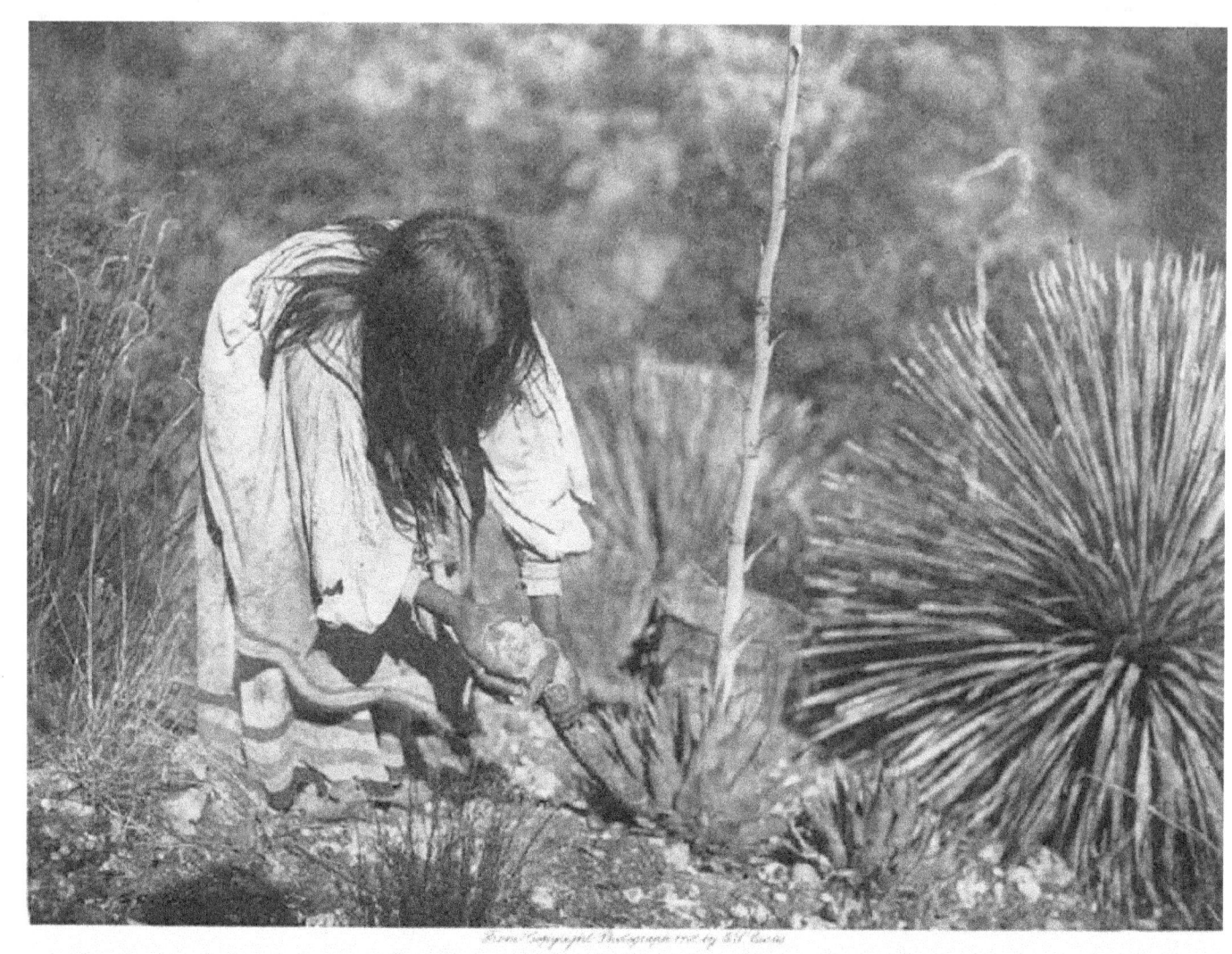

From Copyright Photograph 1906 by E.S. Curtis

CUTTING MESCAL - APACHE

Cutting Mescal - Apache

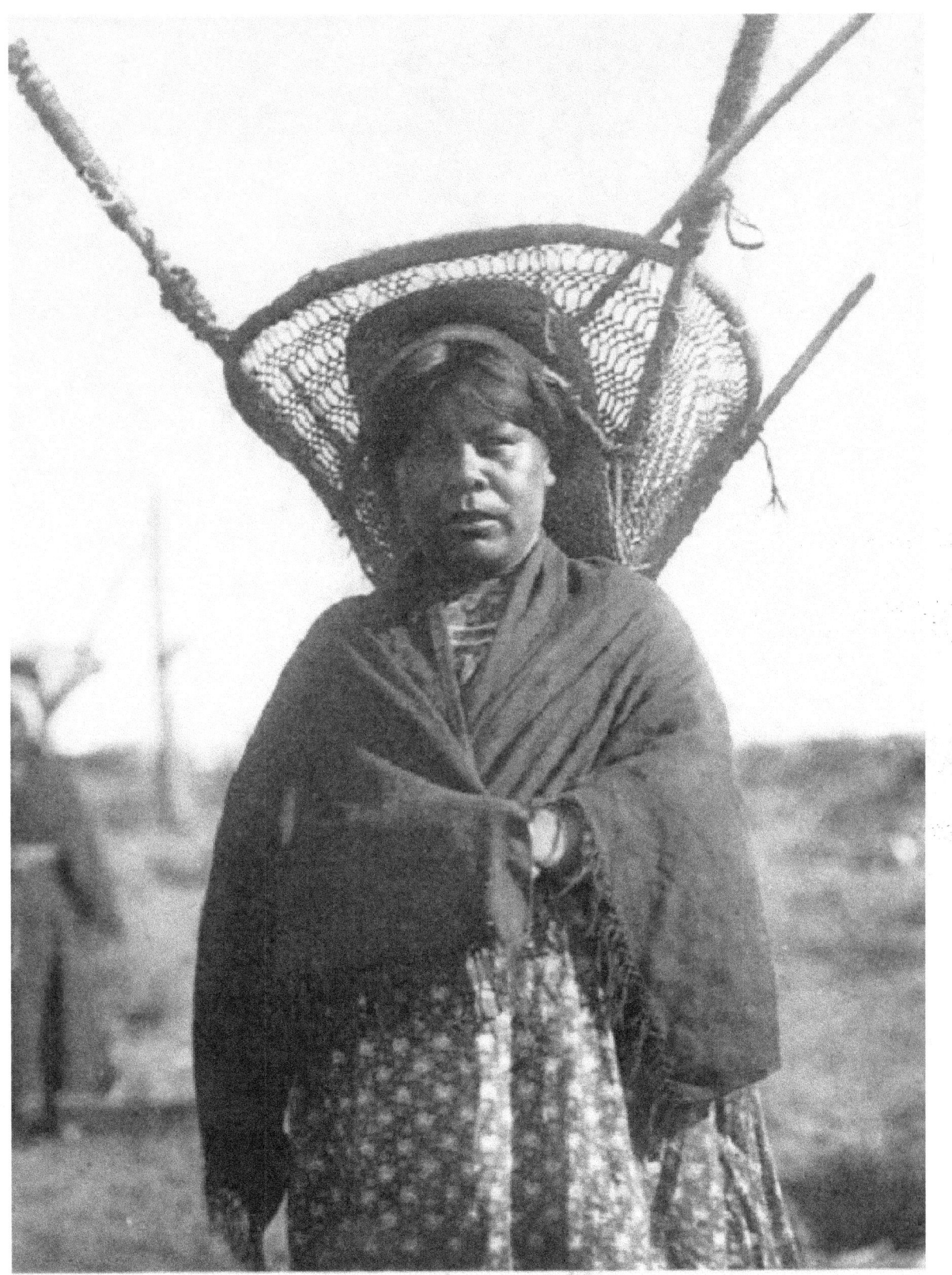

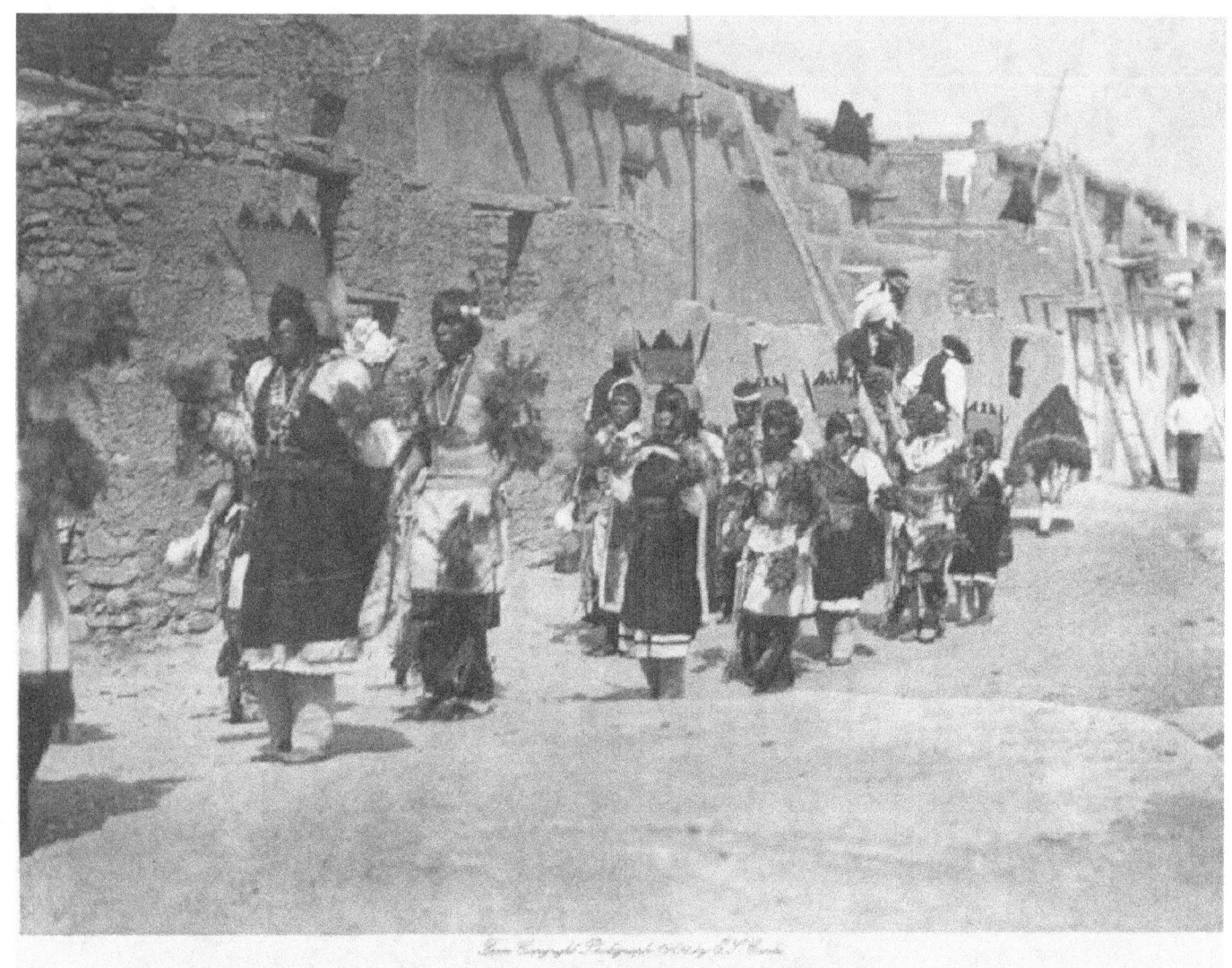

Fiesta of San Estevan - Acoma

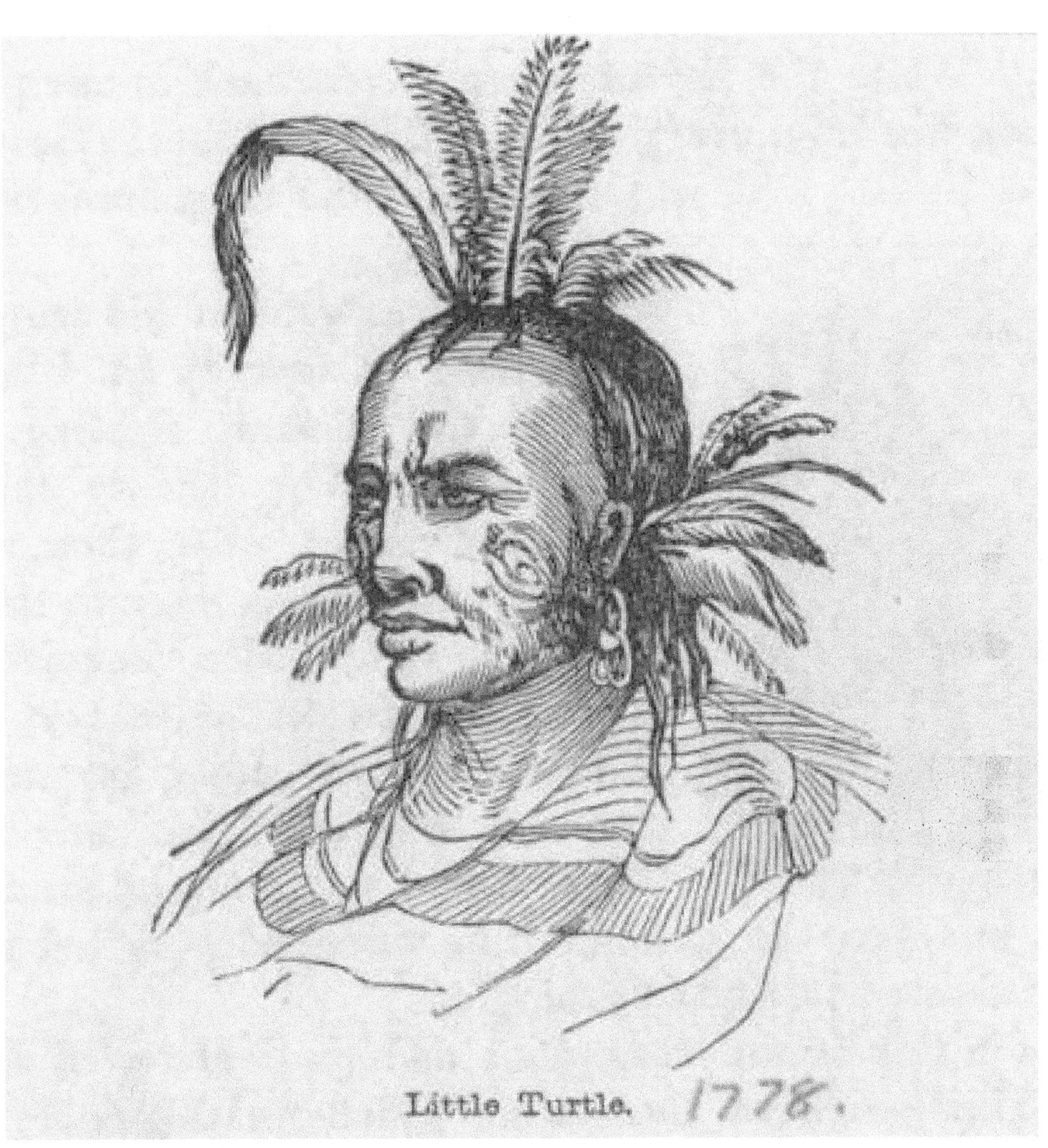

Little Turtle. 1778.

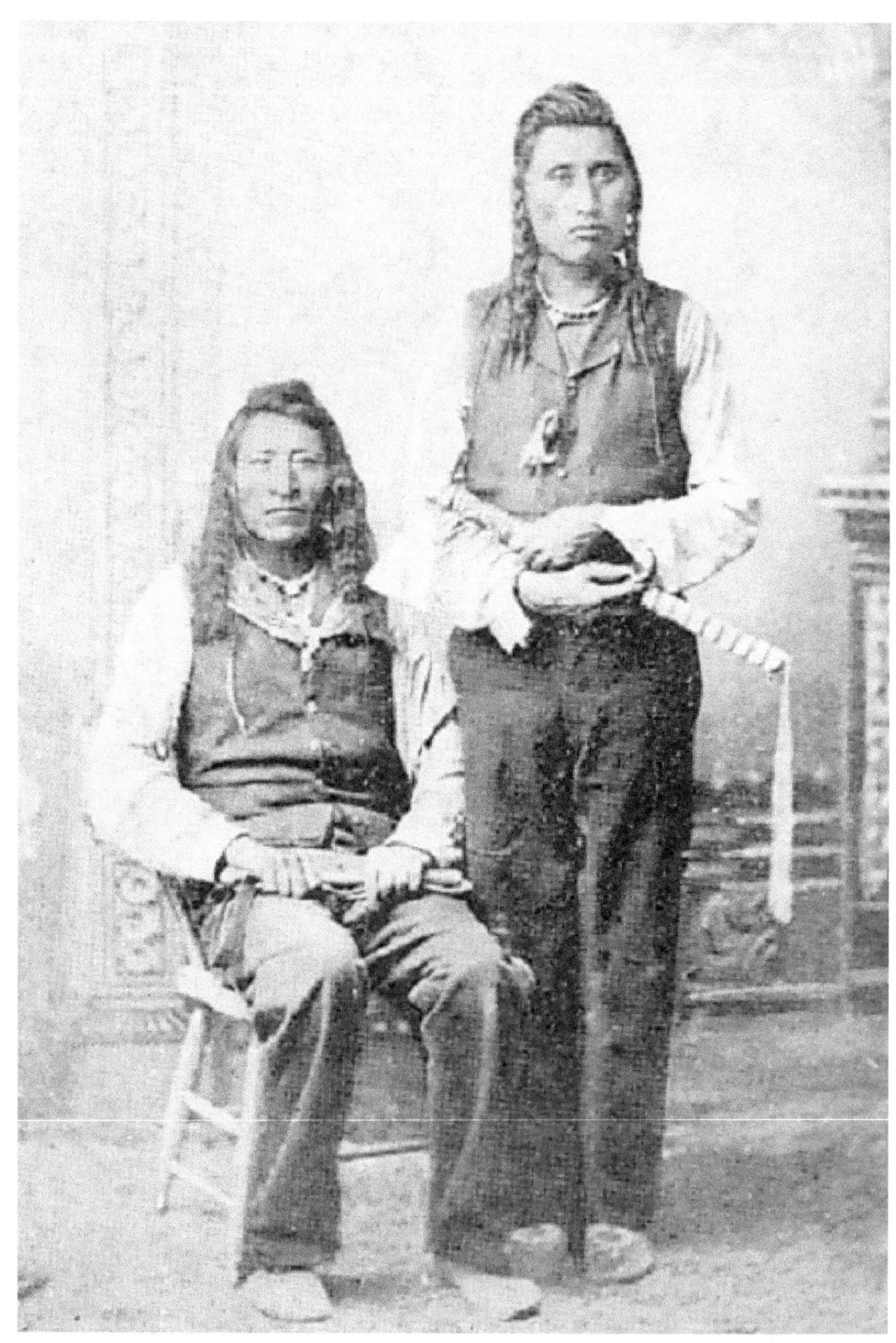

lxxvi

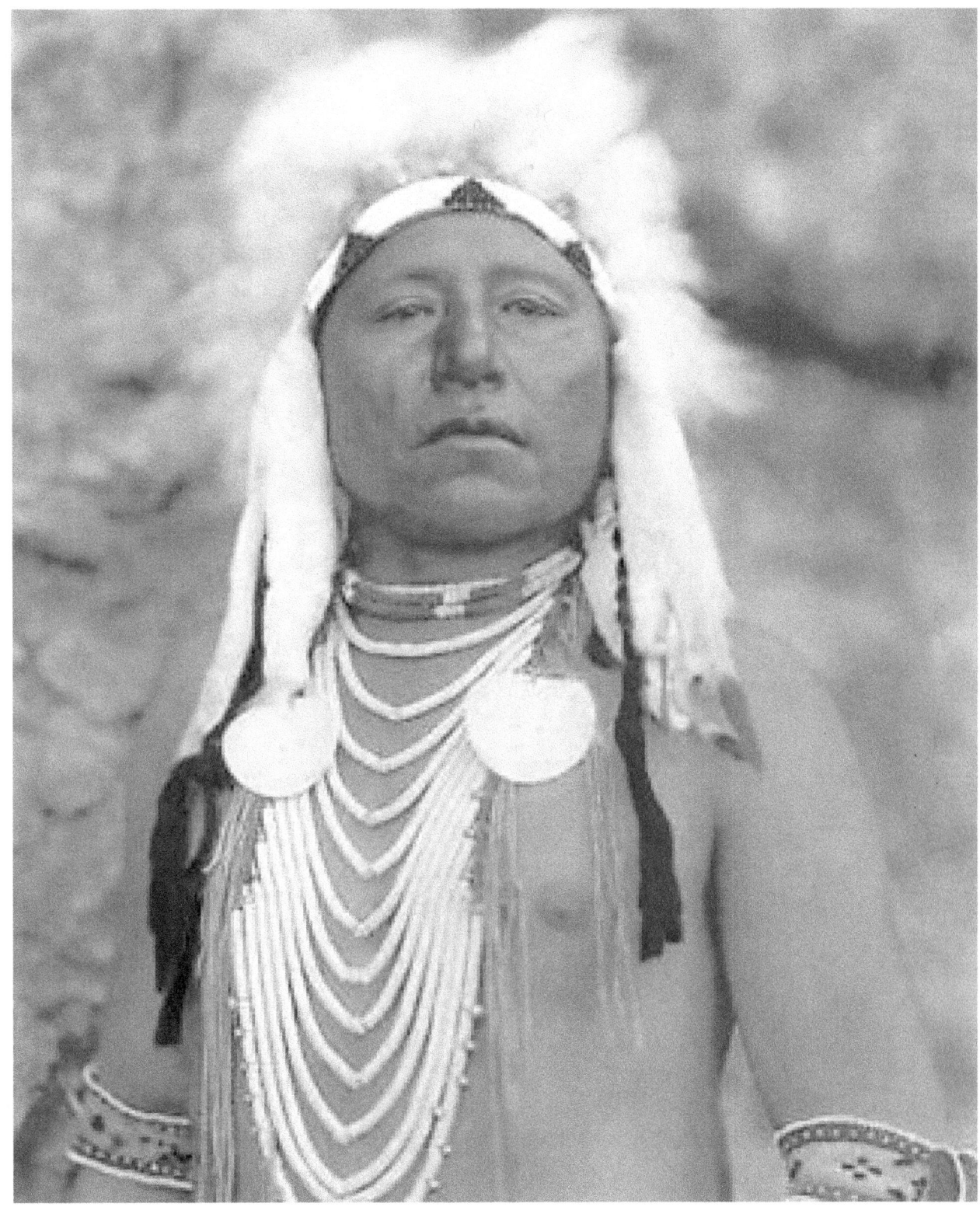

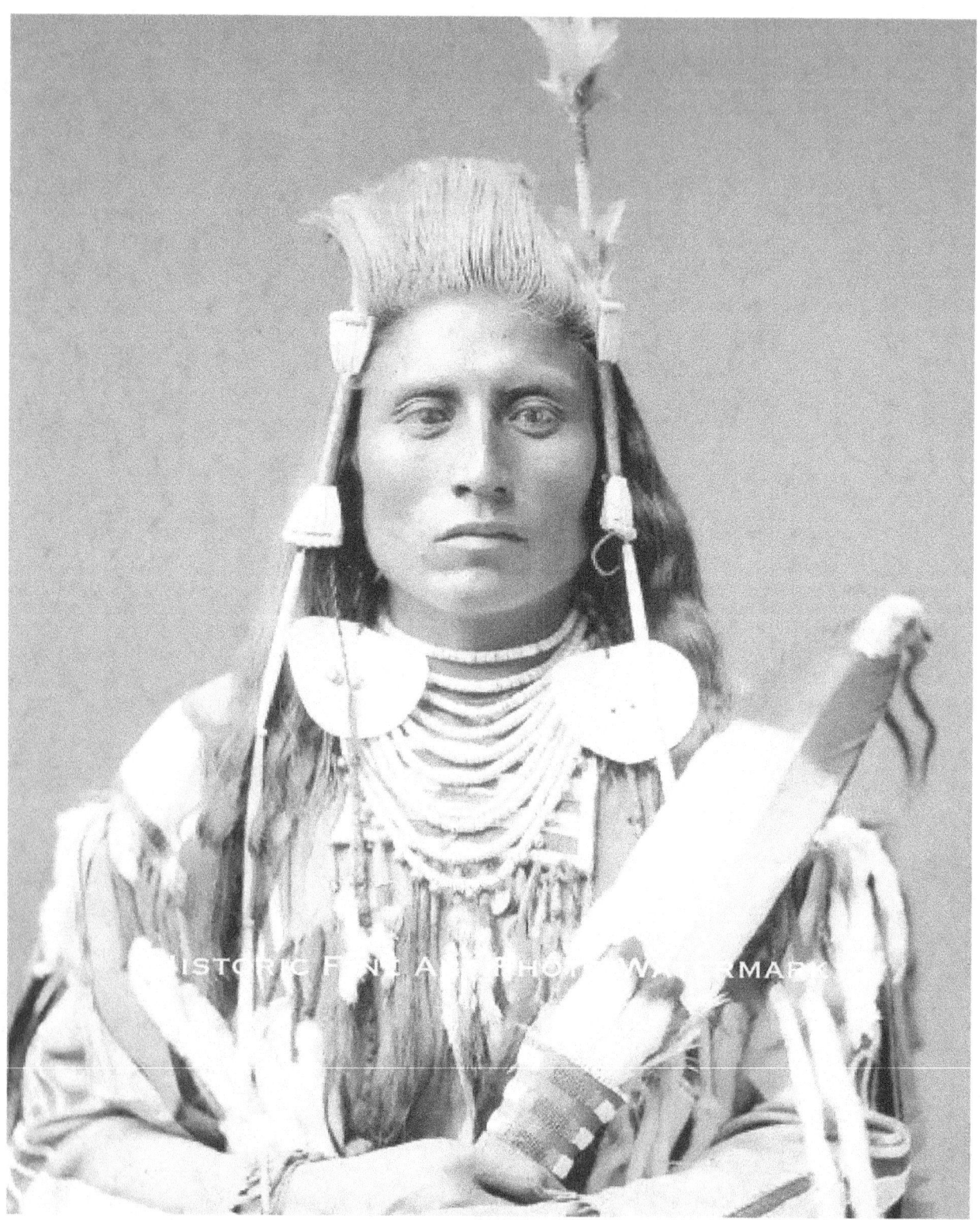

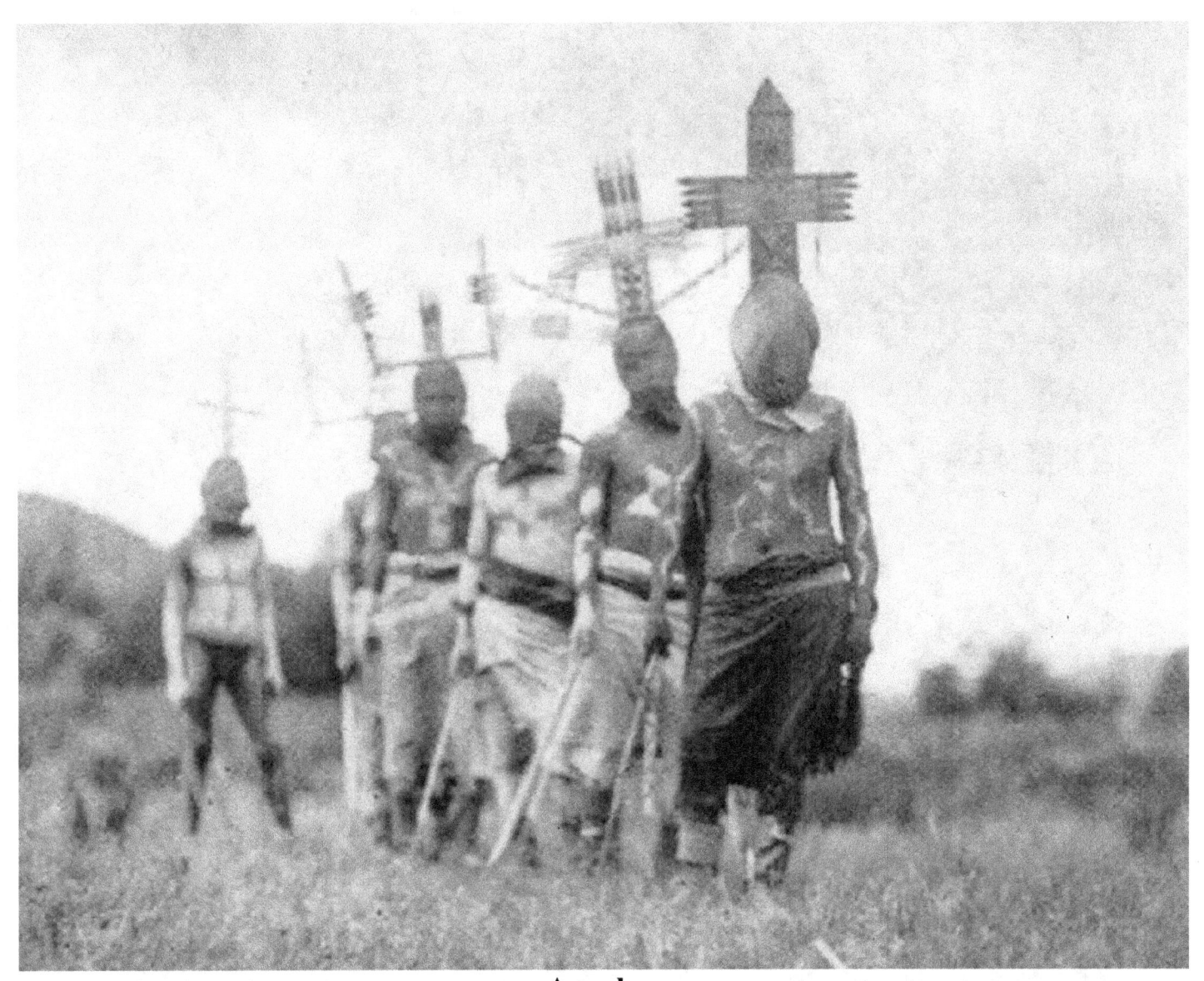

Apache

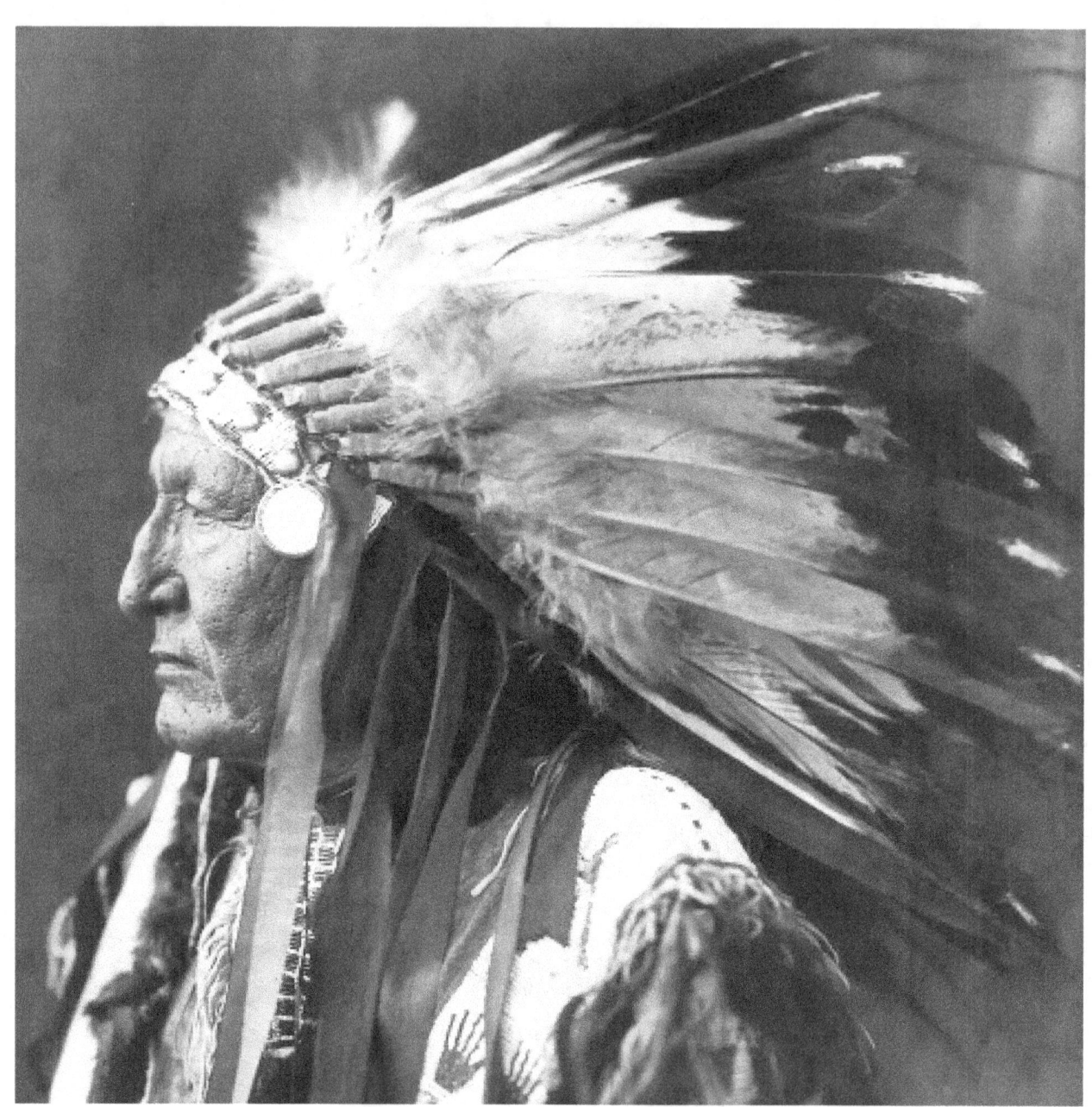

Chief Little Wolf - Cheyenne

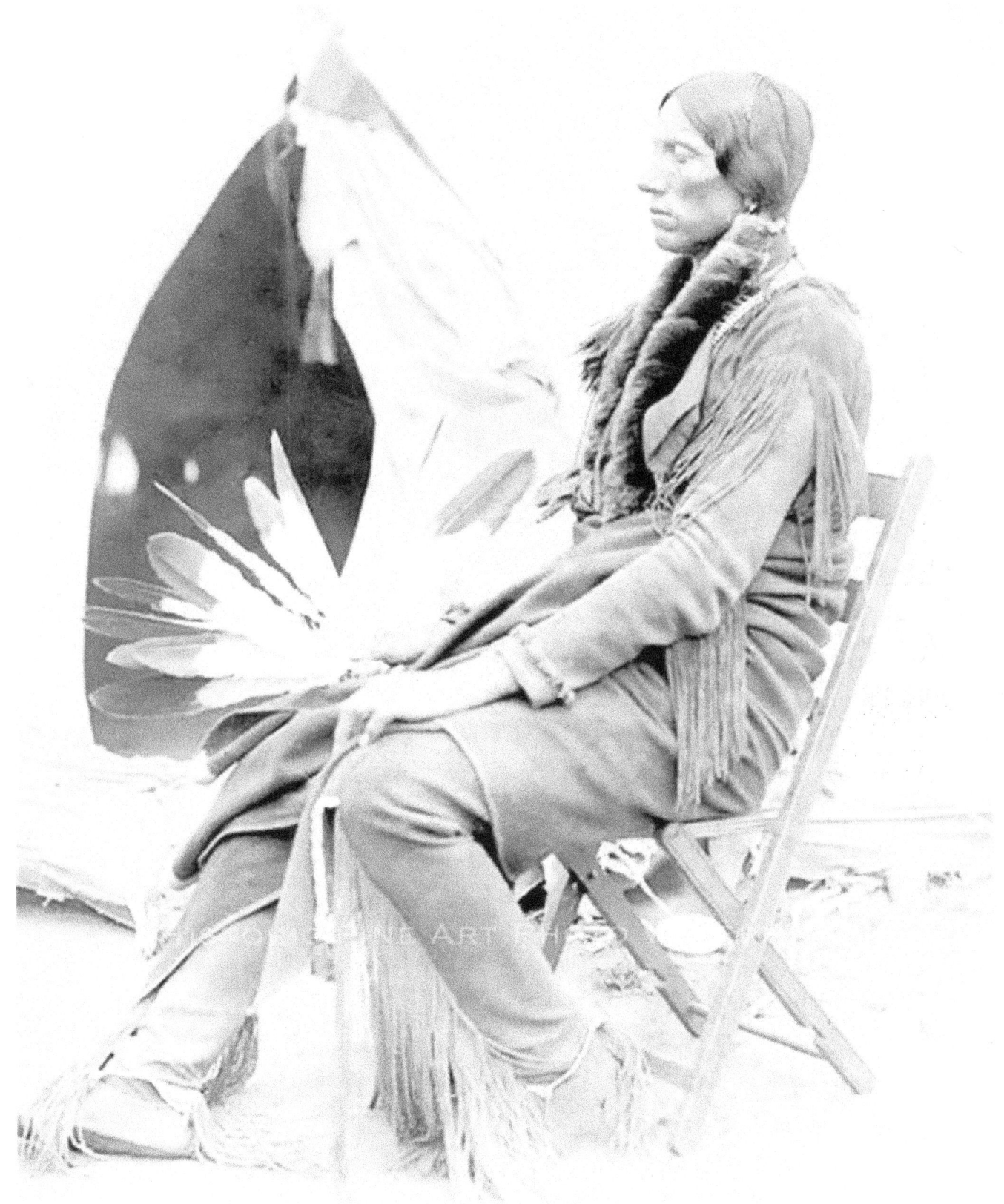

lxxxi

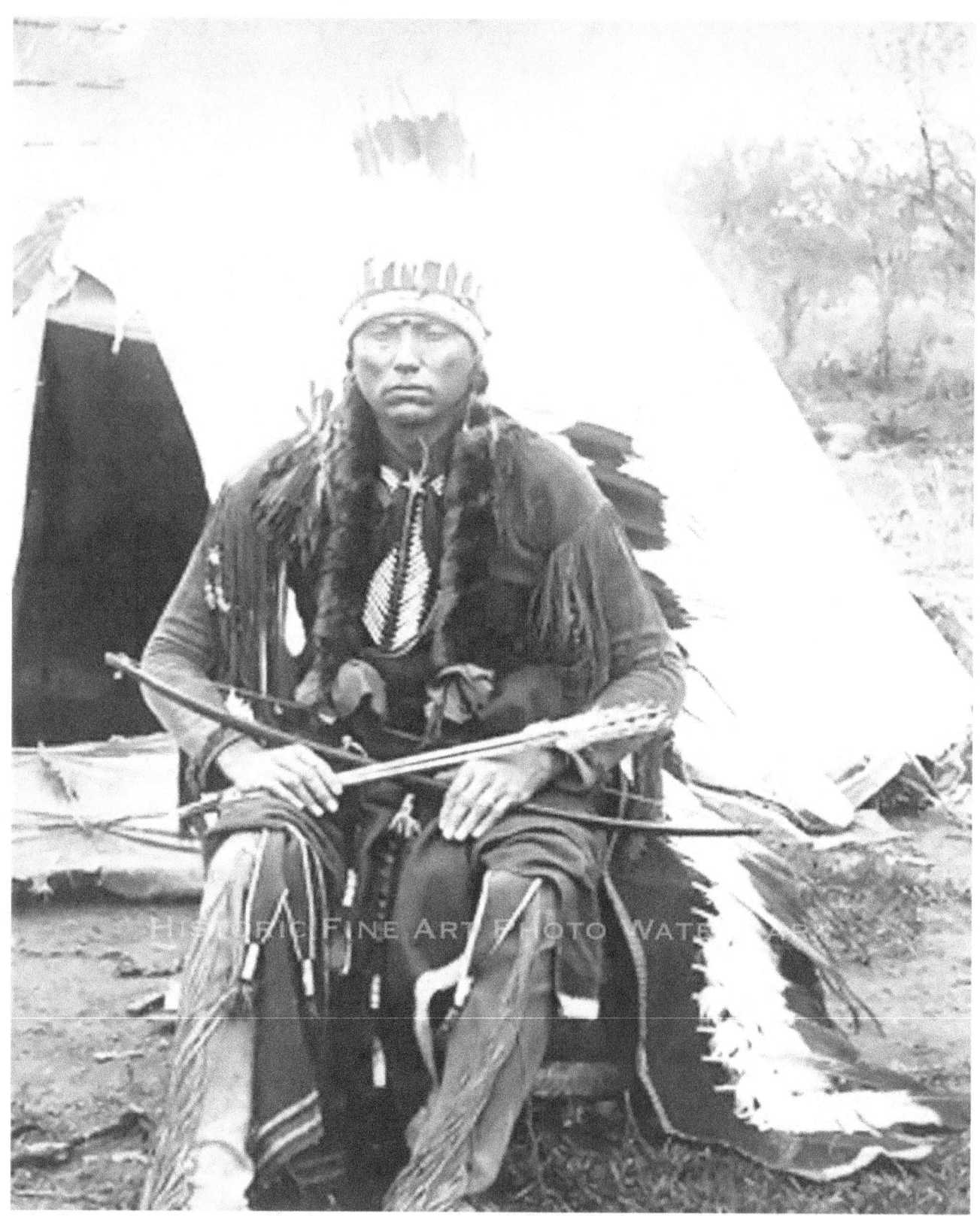

lxxxii

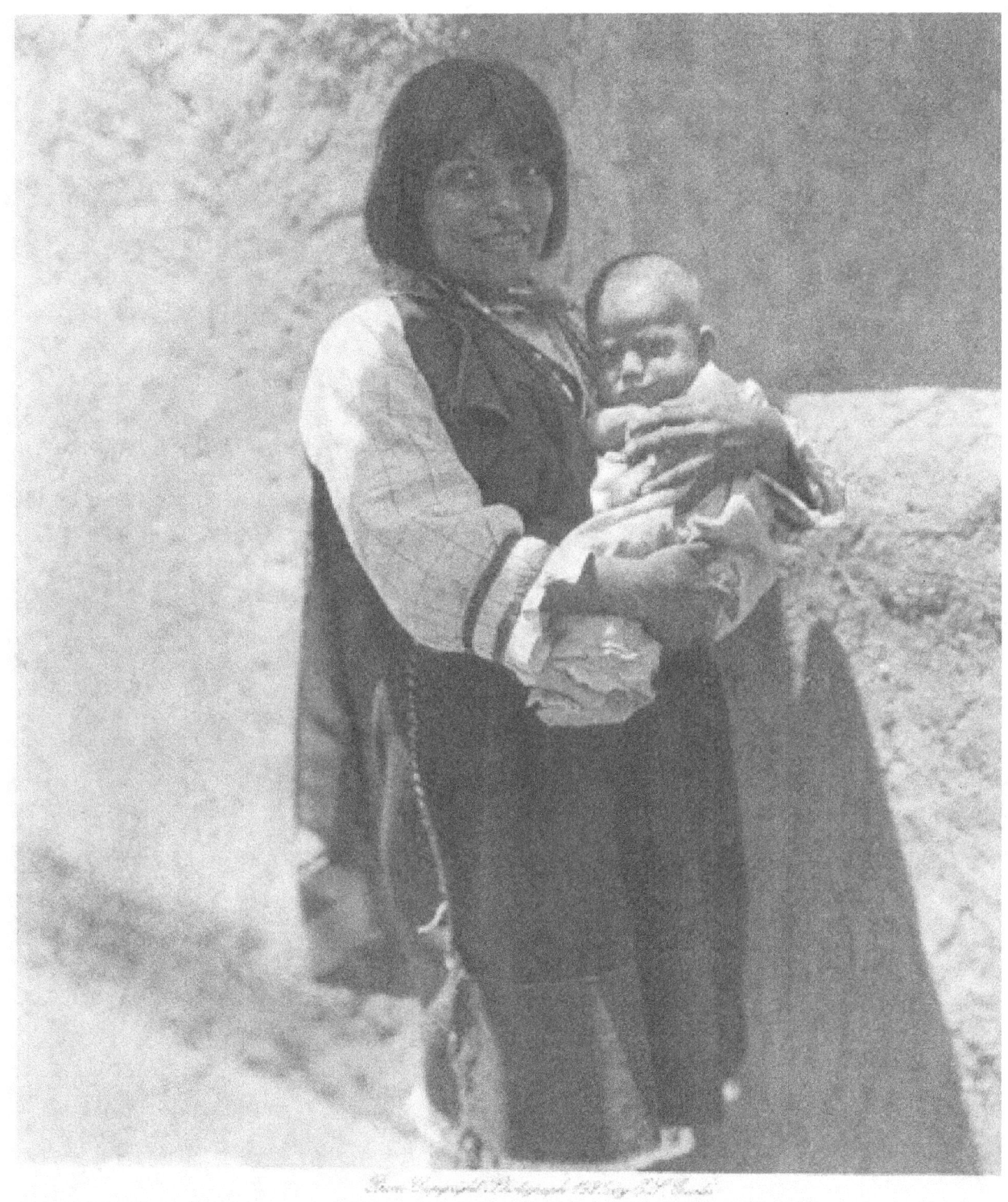

Timu – Cocmiti – 1885, E. L. Curtis

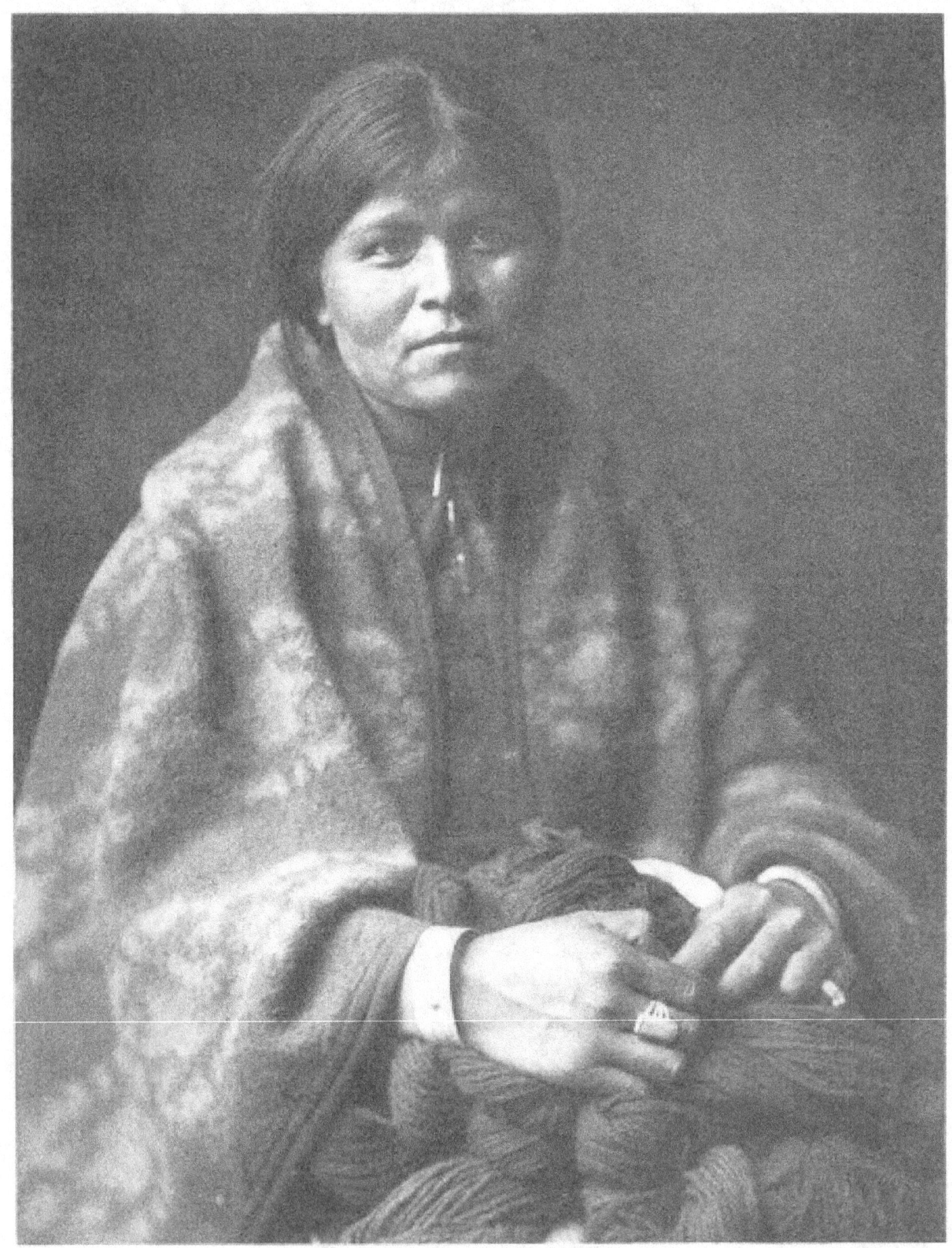

lxxxiv

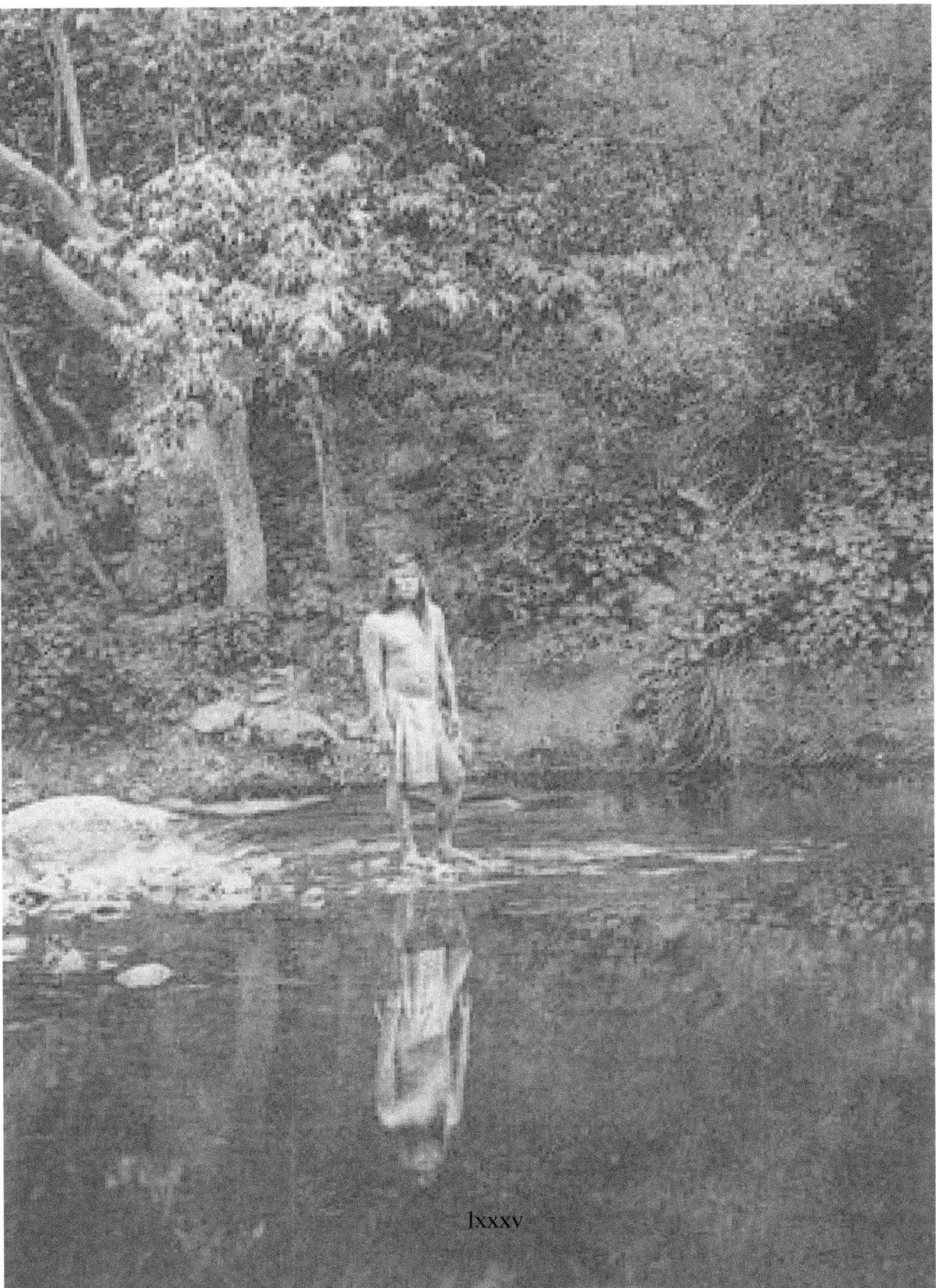

lxxxv

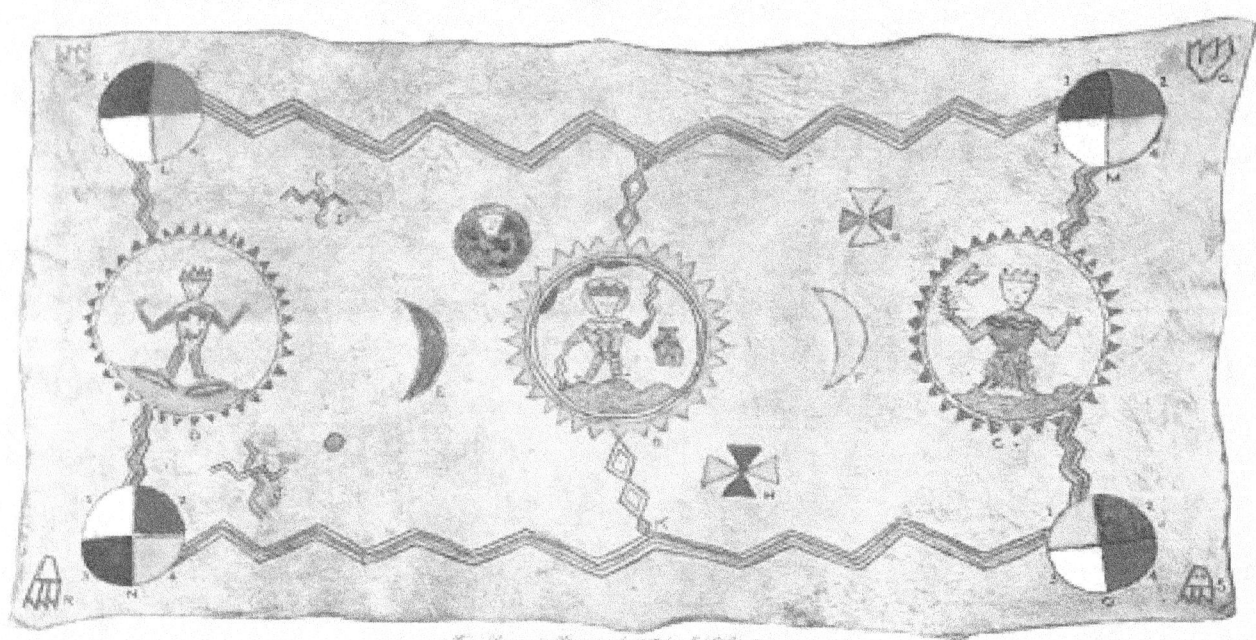

PAINTED BUCKSKIN · APACHE

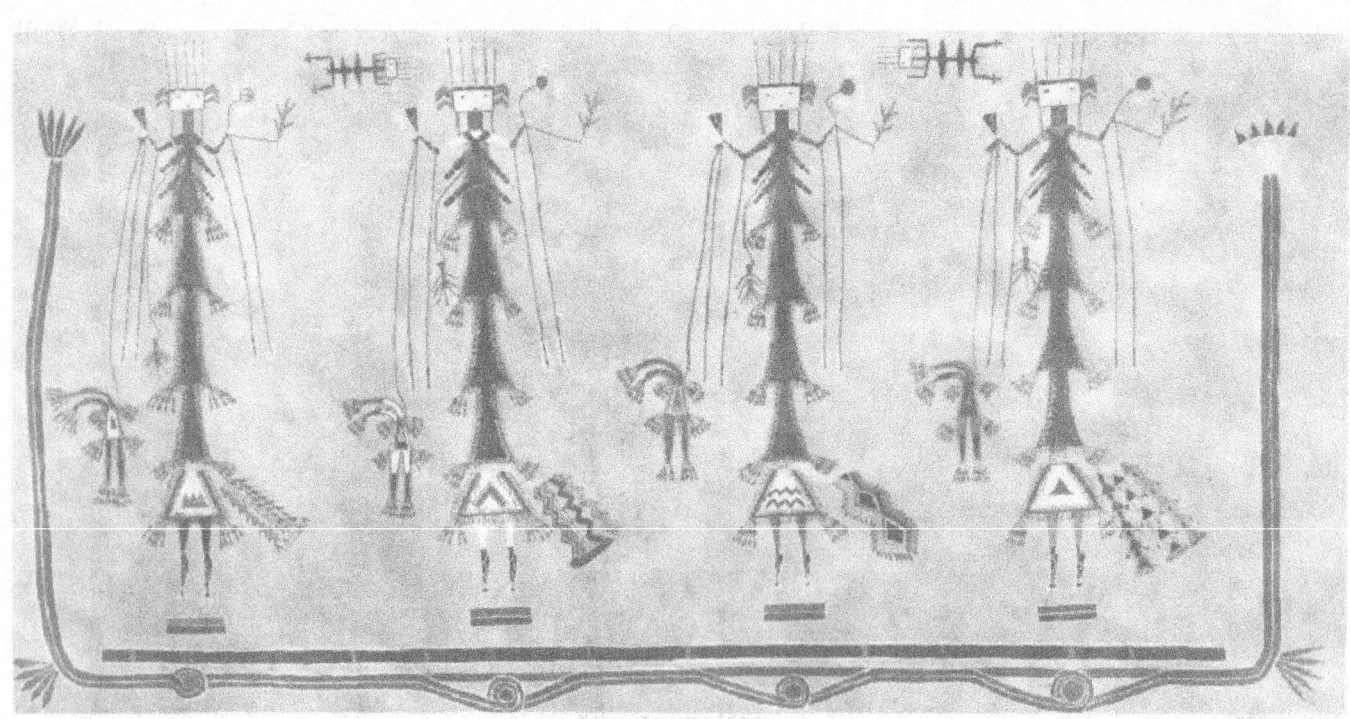

CEREMONIAL RUG · NAVAHO

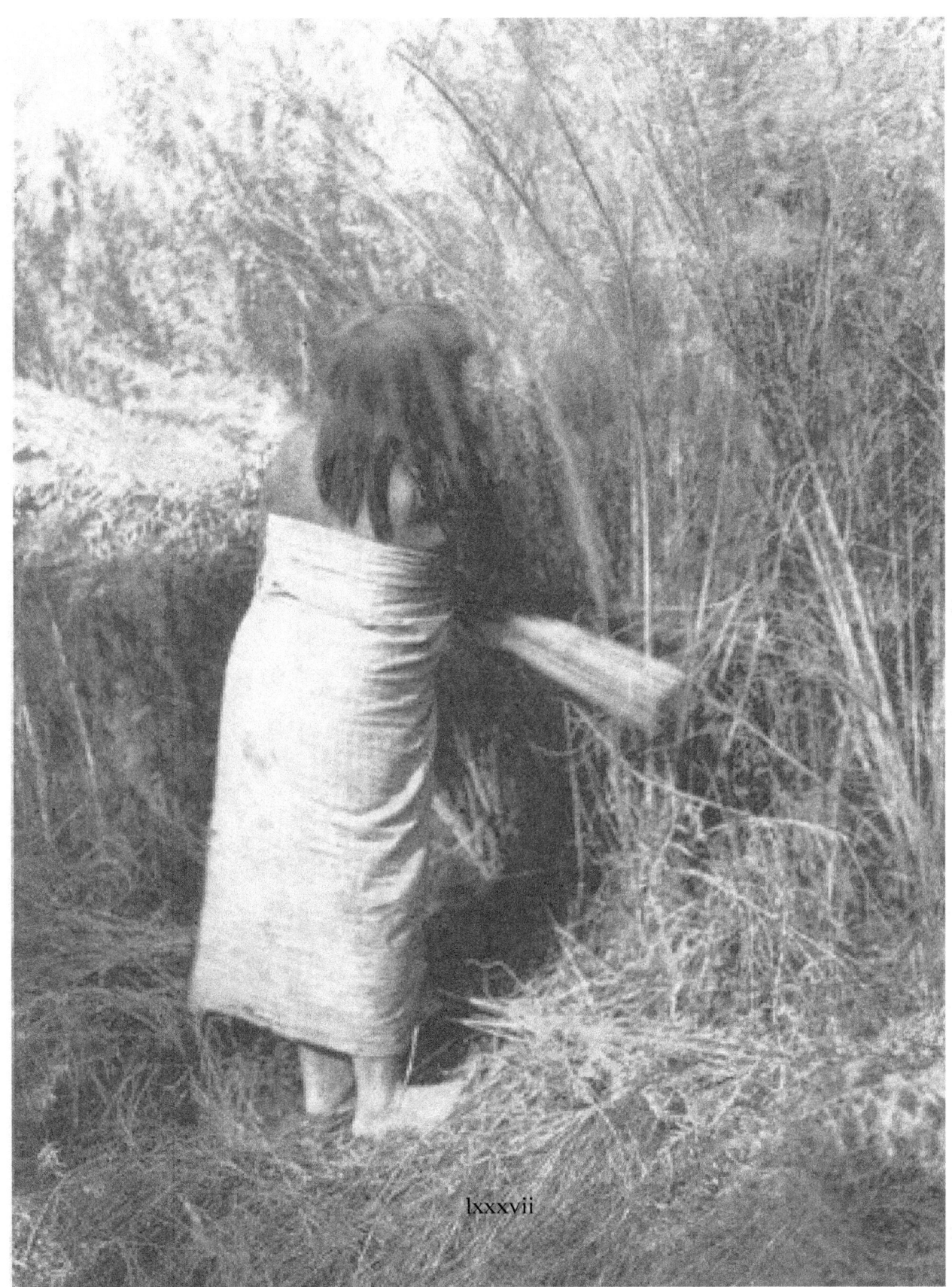

lxxxvii

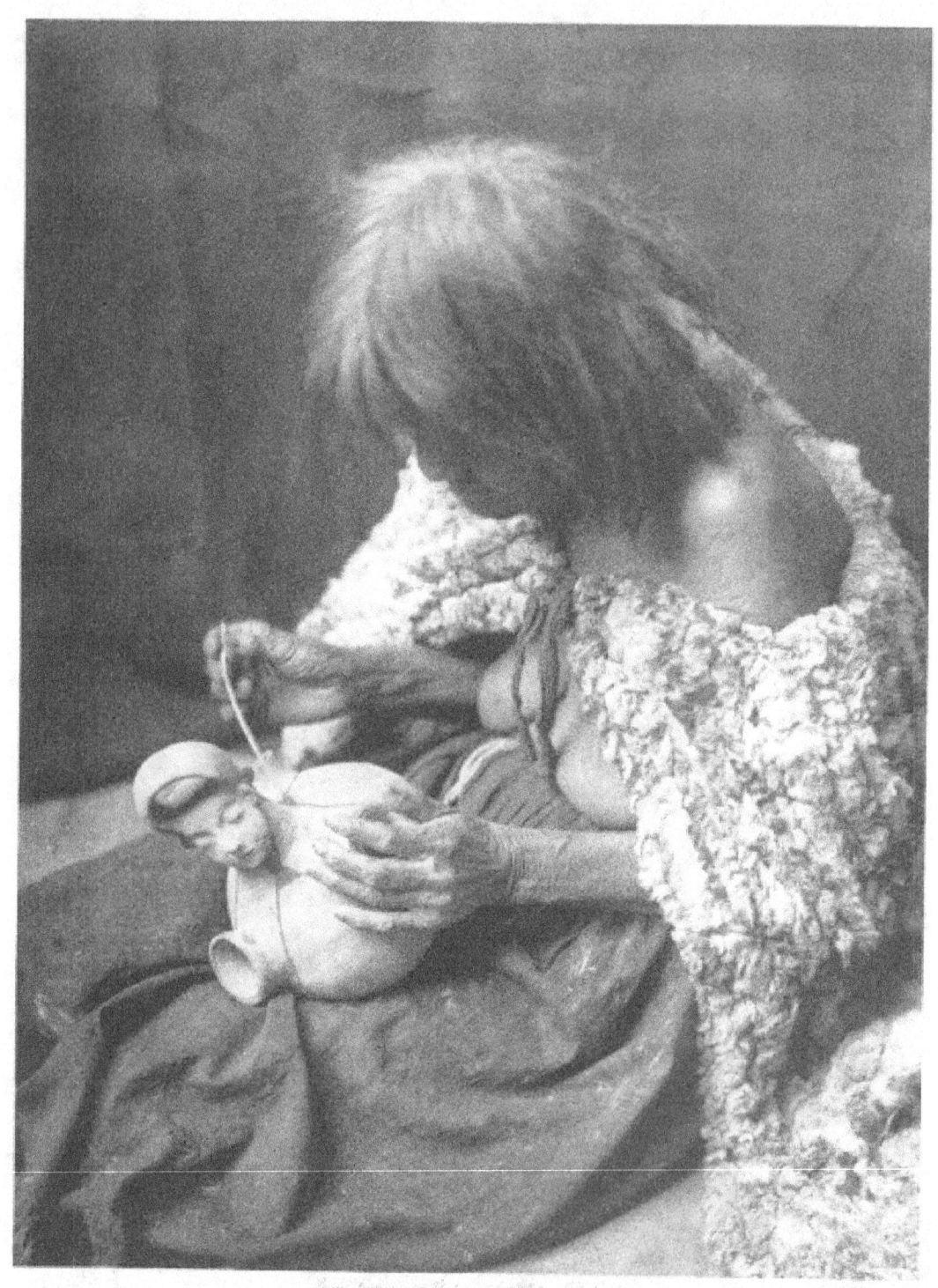

Making Pottery
Good Advice: Lead a life of honor and respect, with the idea of balance in all things.

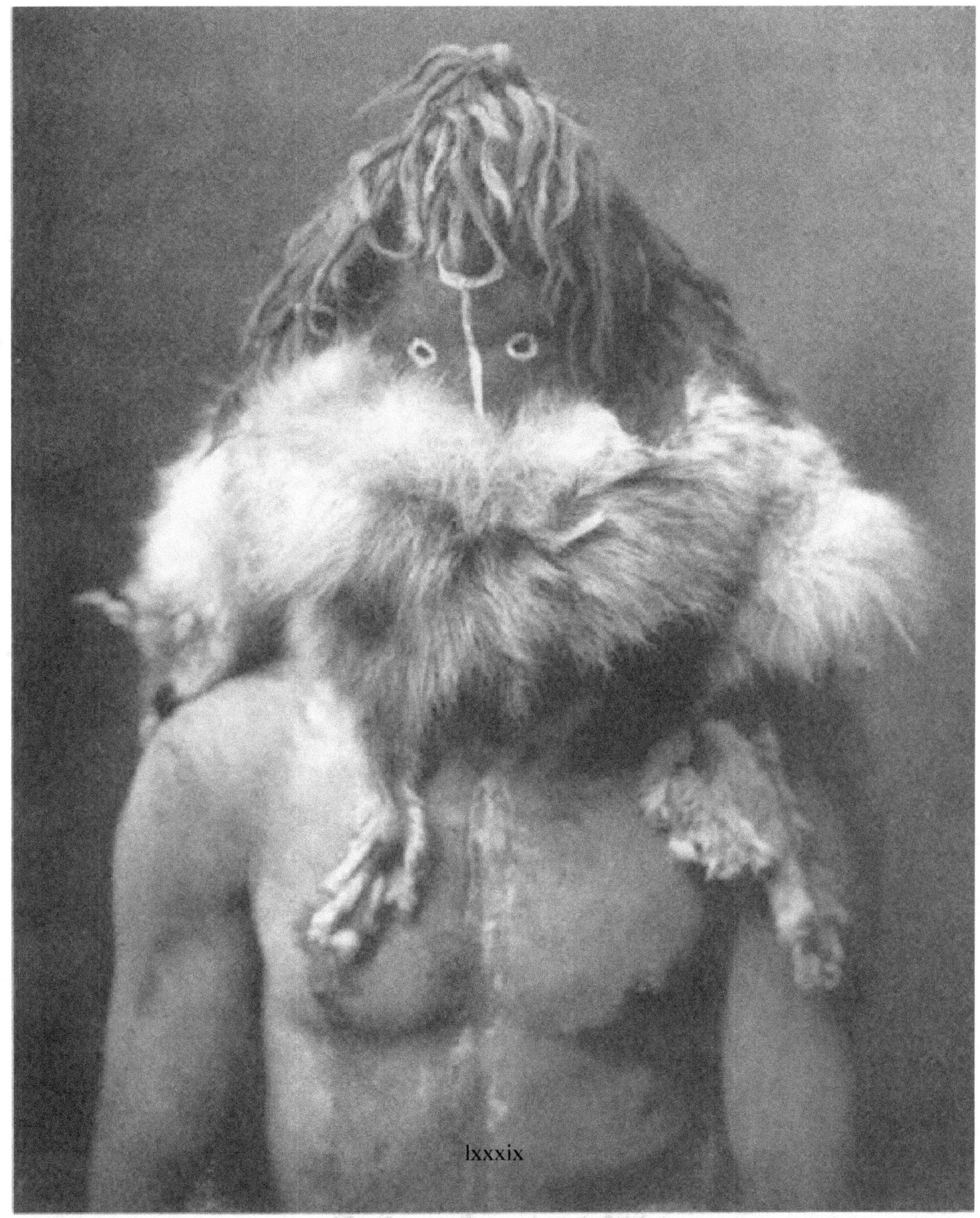

lxxxix

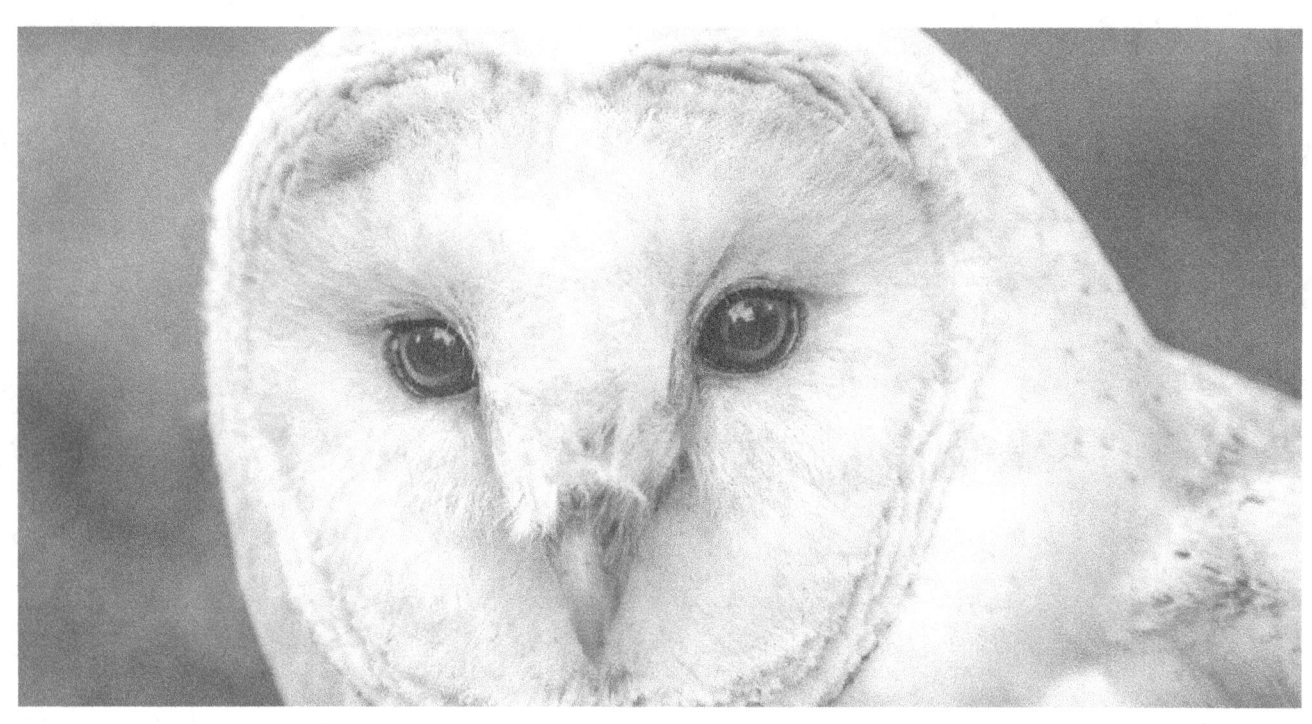

The owl plays a prominent place in Native lore.

This is a Two-Way Communication Process Between the Giver and the Receiver.

Both participants are healed. This is revolutionary. During this process the two participants are healed, and the tribe is also healed. This is truly global healing as one session heals more than one. This is new in the healing field. It still takes time as the trauma can run deep. There can be dialog between the participants, or it can be silent. Healing touch is communication on the kinetic level.

> **Bless You for Being Interested**
>
> **in Your Better Health, and**
>
> **in a Better Healing System.**
>
> **This Book Contains That**
>
> **Blessed Relief of Healing for**
>
> **You and Your Loved Ones.**

The <u>ACE</u> Study, Done by Kaiser Permanente Is Our Medical Validation for The Work We Do. This is Important.

Your lifespan is not entirely determined by your genes. The ACE Study is a thirteen year old study that provides the medical research that validates our hypothesis that early childhood trauma damages our health and longevity. The ACE Study is the scientific medical validation for the healing work that we do. Therefore it is critically important to have individuals do whatever it takes to balance the cell memory of their early trauma.

Just as this study validates our past research in this area, so the fact that past trauma can be unwound, undone, balanced, and neutralized, is a demonstrable fact. This is new information; That you can take responsible control of your health and take action that can vastly improve overall health, and longevity.

Note: This balancing of early trauma is as important as exercise, healthy diet, and healthy life styles. This balancing enhances all your other healthy habits. Keep up your healthy efforts and habits.

We continuously search for medical studies that work, and that were published, but might not have gotten the publicity and wide use that they deserve.
We recently found the "**ACE Study**" done by Kaiser Permanente in cooperation with the U. S. Center for Disease Control and Prevention, (CDC). The initial phase of the ACE Study was conducted at Kaiser Permanente from 1995 to 1997. More than 17,000 participants completed a standardized physical examination. The results of the study were so profound that we would like to share them with you now. This **ACE Study** is the kingpin of our validity for the work that we are doing.

The **ACE Study** had participants fill out a survey of their childhood pains and abuses. From these surveys the data was tabulated, then they correlated this information with later adult illnesses. The results are amazing. The bottom line of this study is; "Tell us of your childhood pain and we will tell you what diseases you may be susceptible to later in life."

Why this is Important to You: From the **ACE Study** survey they can gather information from you and tell you what diseases you may be susceptible to in your later years! **Wow!** The study concluded, and we paraphrase, "Tell us of your early childhood trauma and we will tell you what diseases you will be predisposed to get in your adult years." Important: Can you imagine a study that can be that specific about your future health?

We are so impressed with this **ACE Study** that we are reprinting significant parts of it from the **CDC web site, http://www.cdc.gov/ace/findings.htm**

"Tell us of your early childhood trauma and we will tell you what diseases you will be predisposed to get in your adult years."

- **The ACE Study, by Kaiser Permanente**

All of pages 4, through 6 are directly copied and pasted from this CDC website, they are reprinted with the CDC's permission.

Our continuing message is that one can deliberately and willfully change their health for the better, and even though it takes several hours to do that, you and your loved ones are worth the effort, and you and they are worth the time it takes to undo the trauma of the past.

Your lifespan is partially determined by your genes, the other part is determined by your early childhood trauma. The ACE Study, done by Kaiser Permanente, is a thirteen year old study that provides the medical research that validates our hypothesis that early childhood trauma damages our health and longevity. Our continuing message is that this damage can be reversed, and the negative effects can be eliminated. This is blessed relief for the sufferer, and their families, and tribe.

The (ACE) Study Major Findings
The Adverse Childhood Experiences:

Childhood abuse, neglect, and exposure to other traumatic stressors which we term **Adverse Childhood Experiences** (ACE) are common. Almost two-thirds of our study participants reported at least one **ACE**, and more than one of five reported three or more **ACE**.

The short and long-term outcomes of these childhood exposures include a multitude of health and social problems.

The **ACE Study** uses the **ACE Score**, which is a count of the total number of **ACE** respondents reported. The **ACE Score** is used to assess the total amount of stress during childhood and has demonstrated that as the number of **ACE** increase, the risk for the following health problems increases in a strong and graded fashion:

- **Alcoholism and alcohol abuse**
- **Chronic obstructive pulmonary disease (COPD)**
- **Depression**
- **Fetal death**
- **Health-related quality of life**
- **Illicit drug use**
- **Ischemic heart disease (IHD)**

- **Liver disease**
- **Risk for intimate partner violence**
- **Multiple sexual partners**
- **Sexually transmitted diseases (STDs)**
- **Smoking**
- **Suicide attempts**
- **Unintended pregnancies**
- **Early initiation of smoking**
- **Early initiation of sexual activity**
- **Adolescent pregnancy**

Adverse Childhood Experiences (ACE) Study

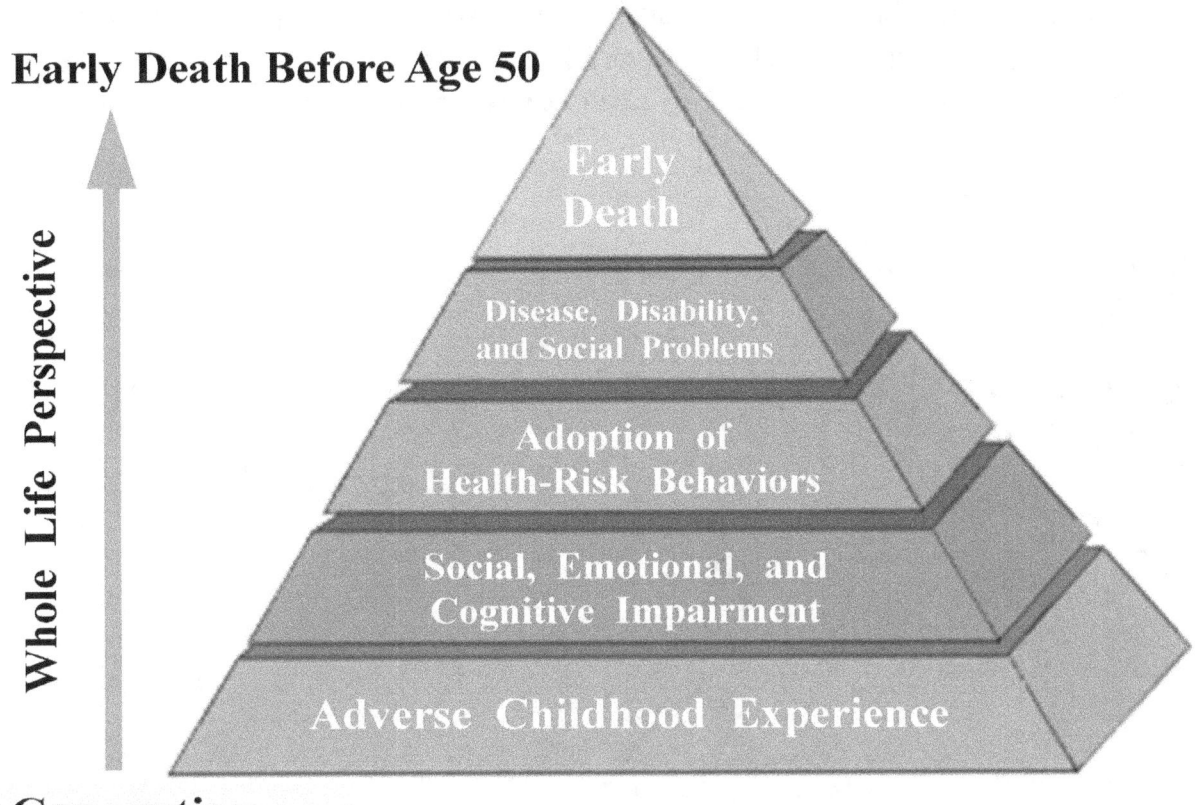

Early Death Before Age 50

Whole Life Perspective

Early Death

Disease, Disability, and Social Problems

Adoption of Health-Risk Behaviors

Social, Emotional, and Cognitive Impairment

Adverse Childhood Experience

Conception

The Adverse Childhood Experiences (ACE) Study is one of the largest investigations ever conducted to assess associations between childhood maltreatment and later-life health and well-being. The study is collaboration between the Centers for Disease Control and Prevention, and Kaiser Permanente's Health Appraisal Clinic in San Diego.

Note: We have enhanced the diagram above for clarity.

More than 17,000 Health Maintenance Organization (HMO) members undergoing a comprehensive physical examination chose to provide detailed information about their childhood experience of abuse, neglect, and family dysfunction. To date, more than 50 scientific articles have been published and more than100 conference and workshop presentations have been made.

The ACE Study findings suggest that certain experiences are major risk factors for the leading causes of illness and death as well as poor quality of life in the United States. Progress in preventing and recovering from the nation's worst health and social problems is likely to benefit from understanding that many of these problems arise as a consequence of adverse childhood experiences.

To contact the CDC:
   Centers for Disease Control and Prevention
   1600 Clifton Rd.
   Atlanta, GA 30333
   (800-232-4636)
   TTY: (888) 232-6348
   cdcinfo@cdc.gov

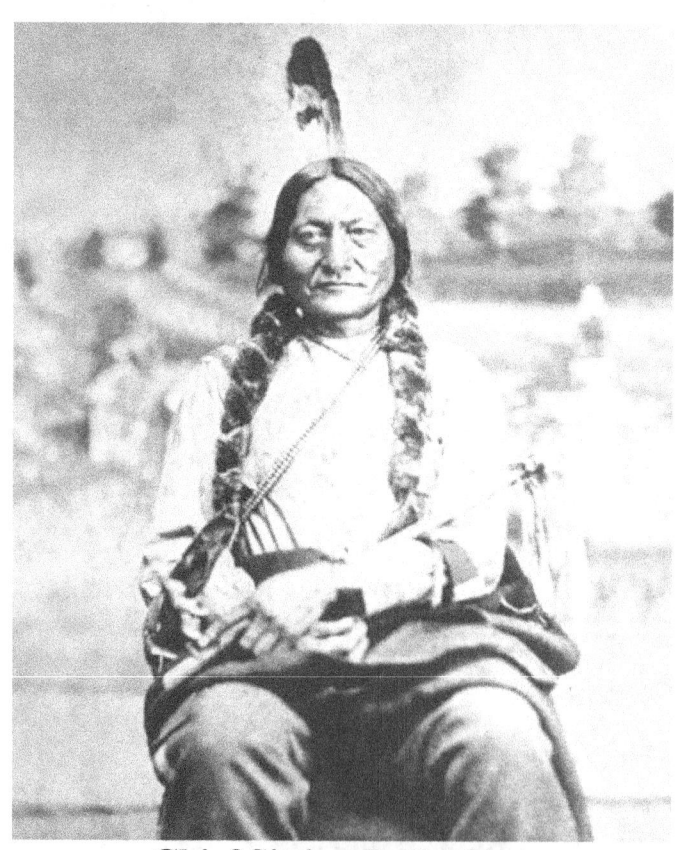

Chief Sitting Bull - Sioux

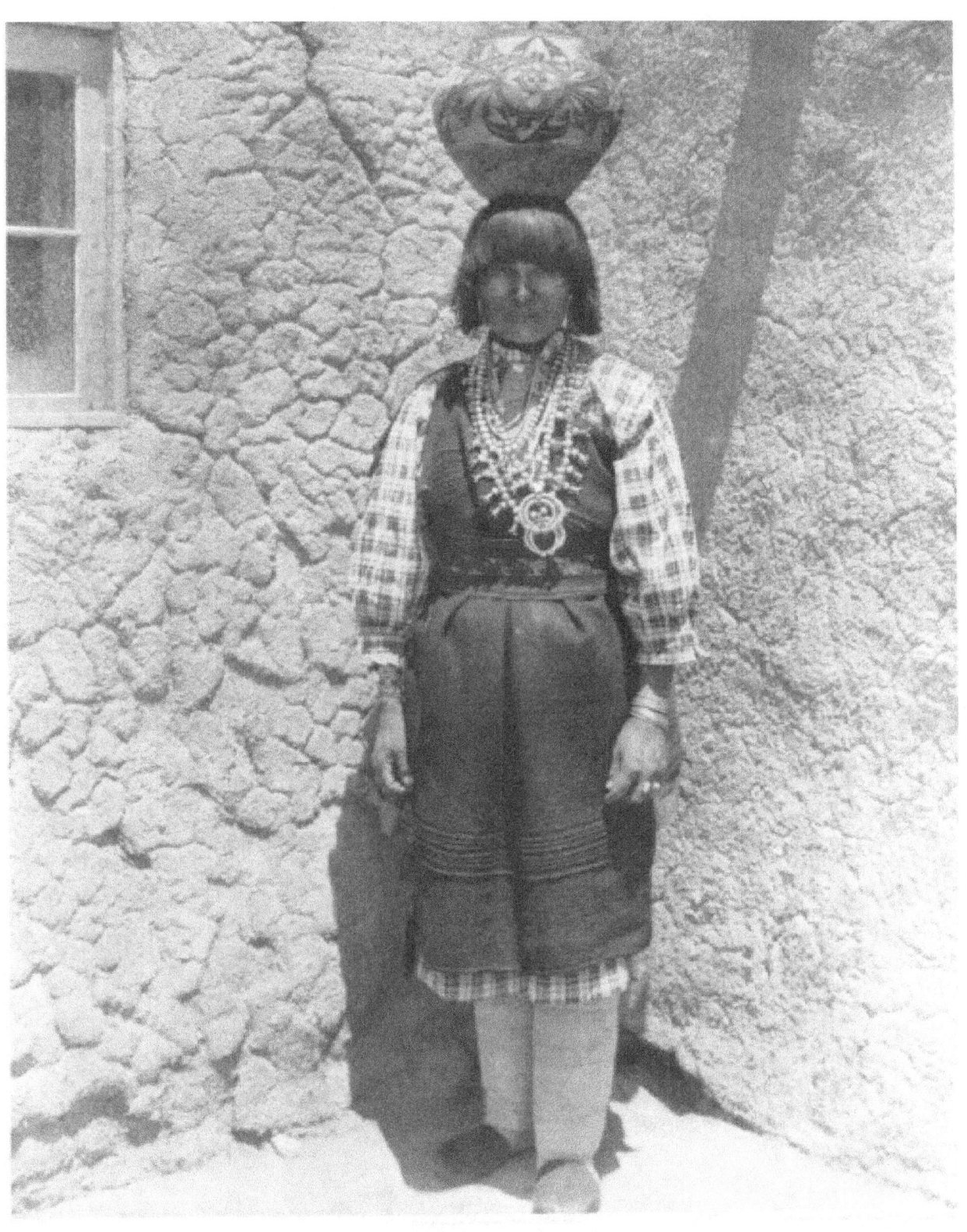

Prove to Me that Cell Memory is Real

About twenty-five years ago a little ten year old girl needed a heart transplant. When another little girl was murdered, the girl on the transplant list got the heart of the dead girl. The transplant girl started having these horrible nightmares of being killed. The parents sent their daughter to a psychiatrist. After months of therapy the psychiatrist concluded that this was not nightmares but recall. This was because the "dream" never changed and the details were vivid. A report was written and sent to the police, the person who did the murder was arrested and convicted on the heart recipient girl's information.

Sends chills down one's spine, doesn't it?

Other transplant recipients who formerly only listened to rap music, start listening to classical music. Others who had no musical talent nor training would, after the transplant, take up playing the piano, flute, violin, or cello. People who had fear of heights would take up extreme rock climbing after a kidney transplant. These stories are searchable on the Internet under "transplant recipient recall."

Comas

This trauma balancing system works well with coma victims. Proof that it is not based upon ones belief system. What would be the benefit if the time in a coma could be cut in half, or by two-thirds? This works because this healing method helps resolve nerve issues. Nerve impulses can flow or be stuck (no flow). It's worth trying.

Note: All healing methods should work to balance stuck energy. The body runs on energy. That energy can flow or be stuck. Balance and flow is better. There is a point where one can feel the balance and flow. There is an energy to it. Creating flow and balance is definitely worth the work.

Energy Explained

Energy is not hard to understand. Albert Einstein was right about energy when he said, "Everything is energy."

Healing can be defined as balance, wholeness, integrity, wellness, and unity (especially within one's own body). When you understand the energy system of your body, the whole world of healing makes sense. The simple way to look at it is that your body is made of energy, and that energy can flow or be stuck. There can be huge amounts of stuck energy in one's body and things still seem to work okay. Future issues can present themselves when the stuck energy is not balanced.

This book shows one how to find the stuck energy and get it to flow. Once the present stuck energy flows, it doesn't stick again, and cannot block itself. That's real healing.

There is no wasted healing. All healing is cumulative, so one healing session builds on earlier sessions. In addition, we all heal together as a whole. One person gets a healing session and others around them get better. Yes! This is true. It's because all of our energy is connected.

What this Means for You!

The good news is that no matter how battered and abused one was as a child, there is a system and a process to balance and reverse the effects of that abuse and physical trauma.

Think of the value of making decisions in present time and not based upon "Pain avoidance at all costs."

Then think of the value of the possibility of adding years or decades to one's lifespan by eliminating the obstacles that compromise ones health. These possibilities exist. As this process is not instant, and as there is a definite time commitment, one needs to arrive at the decision that they are worth the time and effort. Then commit to learning and doing this healing method. Practice makes perfect. There is a "feel" to the method and to peoples energy system.

Balance brings peace and flow to the traumatized cells.
Before now there was no way to "Reset" nor "Delete" nor "Clear" the memory of the trauma from the cells. We have developed a healing system that neutralizes the stuck energy associated with past trauma. This brings balance to your system and promotes healing. This is a gift to you and yours for all of your healing and a better, healthier world.
There are those people in the world who make money keeping people sick and strung out. They may not like a system that actually works. We need to deal with that hurdle when it presents itself.

How Pain Works in the Body

This is all new information and it is true: The memory of pain is cumulative in the cells. The earliest pain empowers later pain just like the cells in a battery. Enough pain over time and the pain becomes self generating and chronic. Our continuing message is that there is a process to undo this early pain. That gives blessed relief to the sufferer. The proof is in the doing of the process.

It can take hours but you and your loved ones are worth it.

The PYRAMID of PAIN

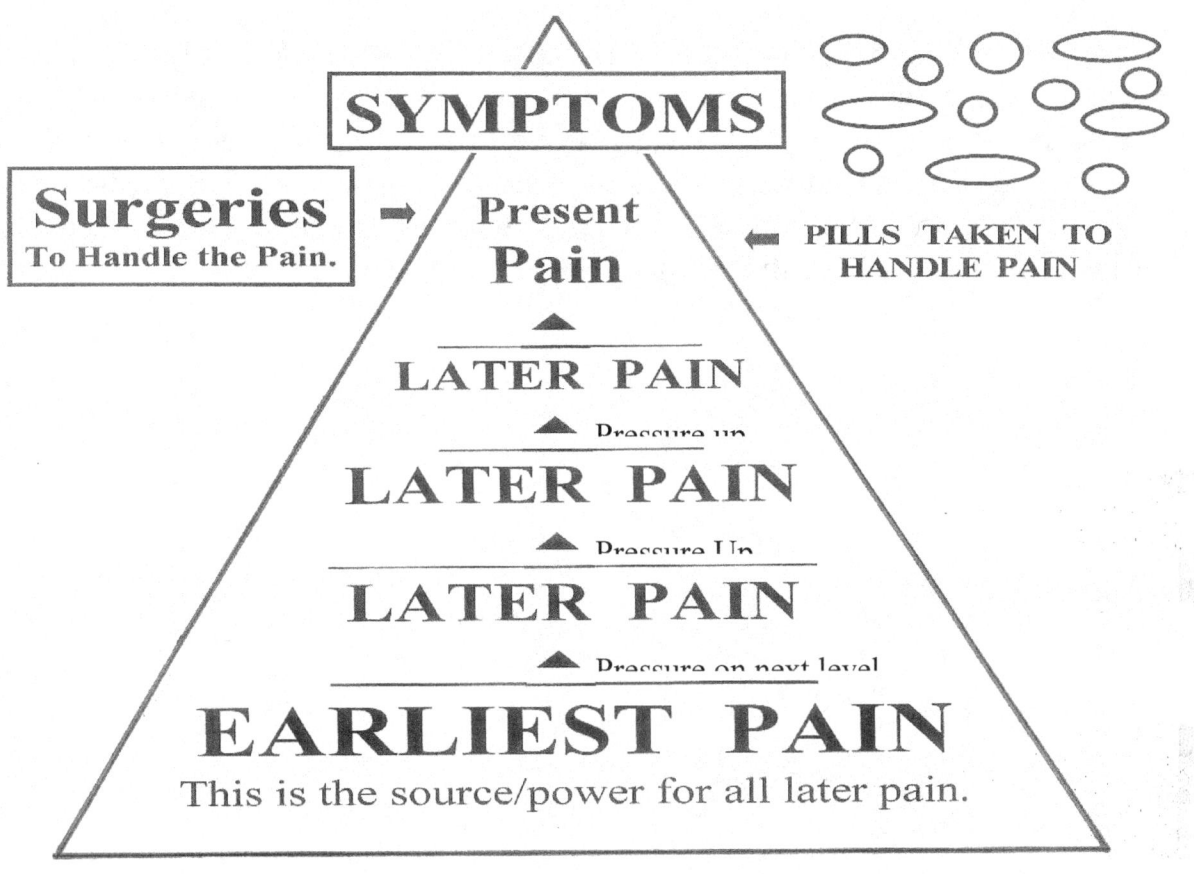

SYMPTOMS

Surgeries
To Handle the Pain.   →   Present
Pain   ←   PILLS TAKEN TO
HANDLE PAIN

LATER PAIN

Pressure up

LATER PAIN

Pressure Up

LATER PAIN

Pressure on next level

EARLIEST PAIN
This is the source/power for all later pain.

This diagram is read from the bottom to the top.

Notice: Each lower level produces pressure on the level above it much like a geyser.

Pain is cumulative. Healing is cumulative, also. The Pyramid of Pain shows how pain develops in the body. The upward arrows in the center of the pyramid indicate that the earliest layer of pain produces pressure on the next level up. After many years of pain building up, chronic pain is energized, empowered and manifests. It is the earlier and earliest pain that energizes the present pain. Please also notice that pills, drugs and surgeries can not do anything to fix or balance the earliest/original pain. What if there was a system that gets to the root cause and could reduce the effect of early childhood trauma to zero? The good news is that there is a simple process to resolve early trauma from the past. This restores balance and flow to the energy systems of the body. The

11

body knows how to heal itself when the energy blocks are removed. This is new and revolutionary. This is very real. The results speak for themselves. The key is in doing this process with love and patience. Working together for a healing result.

Note: The entire medical profession exists at the top of this Pyramid of Pain. That is the chasing of symptoms with pills and surgeries. We need a different and better healing model. We are not the "plankton" to be "practiced on" that some think we are. Healing is as much a spiritual process as it is a physical one. The value of healing one's spiritual issues is tremendous and can not be overstated. Forgiveness also is a part of healing as it is part of the spirit.

The Remedy of Pain's Energy System

Using the 1 – 2 - 3 Process the source of pain is gone!
This is a first. A process like this has not existed before now!

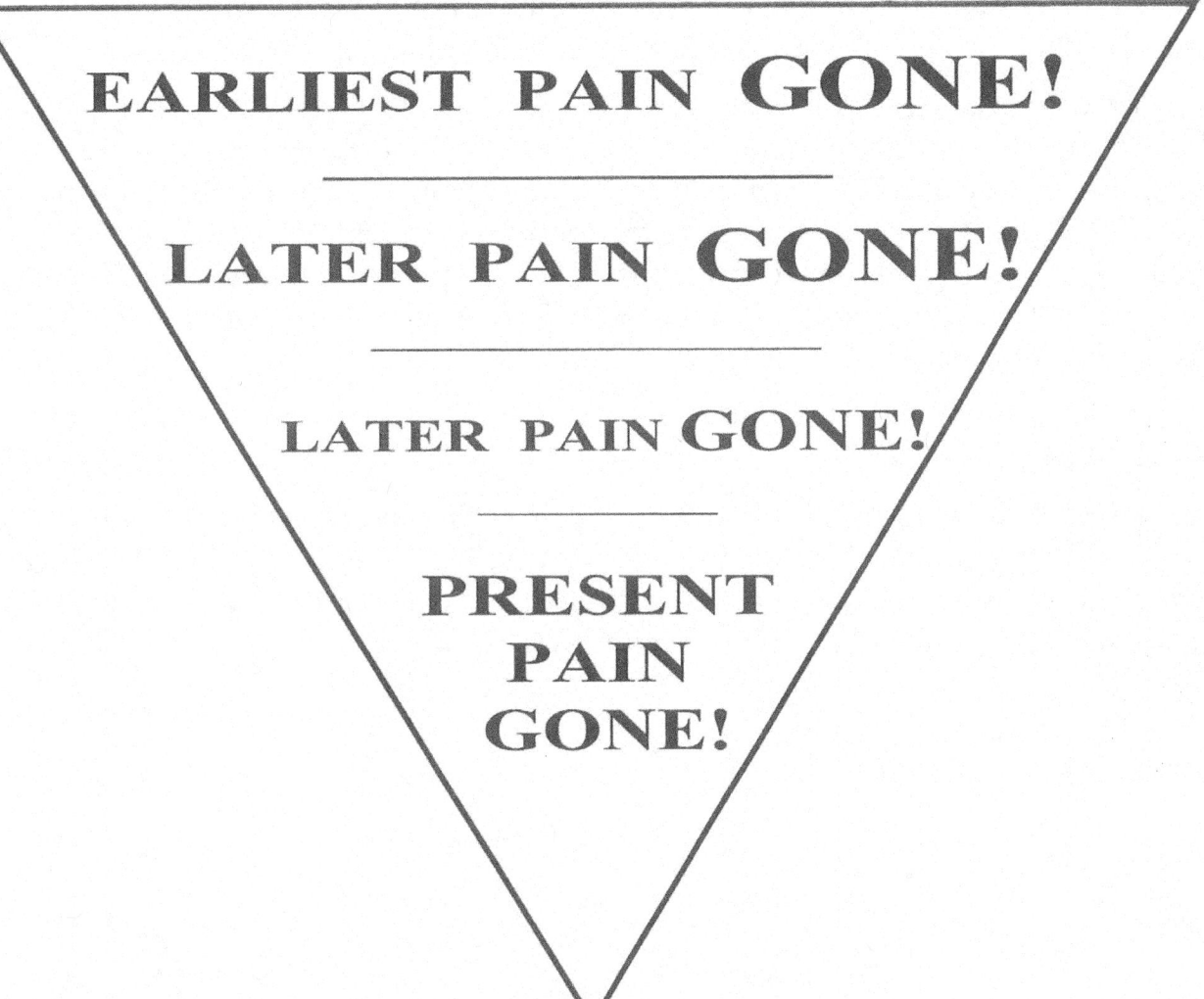

Please Study this Remedy of Pain's Energy System.

Please note that the source of pain is gone. Does it make sense that pills and surgeries do not remedy/balance the earliest pain? Does it make sense that only handling the earliest trauma resolves later pain?

What do you suppose would happen if all early trauma was balanced before chronic pain or disease set in?

Can you fathom the possibilities of Kaiser's **"ACE Study"** being scientifically correct?

Please notice that the symptoms, the pills, and the original source of the pain is gone! There is a simple system that resolves pain and trauma from the past.

The proof of this process is in just doing it and getting results. When we know what and where pain is coming from, and we know how to neutralize that source using this method, handling pain becomes relatively easy. It does require practice and patients because it takes as long as it takes and every body is different. Rome was not built in a day, and your health was not compromised in a day. This method takes work and commitment. The results, and you and your tribe are very much worth the work and the commitment.

This system also handles past emotional pain, such as PTSD, and other stress and nerve-related issues.

This system also works well even during a coma. That is the proof that this process works at the cellular level and repairs traumatized nervous systems. Balancing the nervous system restores nerve communication and vastly improves all the functions of the body including digestion and the immune system functions.

Past Model for Handling Pain –

Chasing Symptoms with Pills!

In the past handling pain was the "Symptom-pill, symptom-pill, symptom-pill model" with the discouraging and suspicious results of the medications eventually producing symptoms of their own, necessitating more pills to handle those new pill-generated symptoms.

The wonder and amazement of this "chasing symptoms with pills" system of medicine is that the greatest thinking minds in all of history didn't see anything wrong with this model. The symptom isn't where the pain is coming from. Pills may handle symptoms, but pills don't and can't handle the source of the pain.

Just think for a moment, what could change in a person's life if the original source of pain was eliminated, and a healing model was built on keeping people strong and healthy? Isn't it about time that suffering people are given some relief?

Pain-Anchored Life Decisions

The effort to avoid pain and painful experiences causes many people to make life decisions based on pain avoidance at all costs. Sometimes these decisions are made as a young child, with little ability to think of possible future consequences. These are called "pain-anchored life decisions."

All future decisions are then made through this pain avoidance filter. A person's life may not go well and decisions may not work, or work poorly, because this template for making decisions is so skewed and not relevant to the present time. The past pain, therefore, influences all one's future life decisions. This can cause "crash and burn" decisions. This is why early childhood abuse is so destructive for the whole rest of a person's life from the time of the injury.

The symptom isn't where the pain is coming from. The pills may handle the symptoms, but pills can't and don't handle the source of the pain and may produce symptoms of their own. For the first time we now have a system for eliminating the source of the pain – naturally, without chemicals nor drugs. This is great news for all pain sufferers.

Silver Bullets and Magic Pills

These processes are not instant. There are no magic bullets. There are no magic pills.

As Rome was not built in a day, and as your immune system was not instantly compromised, so these processes take time and work to achieve long lasting results. You and your partner are worth the work. You both are worth the time spent, and you are both worth working toward the results and outcomes of balanced energy and flow.

No claims of results can ever be made from these processes because every body and every trauma is different, and heals differently. Some chronic pain does not respond to balanced energy, one is always free to explore other avenues of healing.

Just for clarity, there is no suggestion that there is anything wrong with the reader, their families nor friends, nor any of our societies. We are all made perfectly. There is nothing wrong with you or anyone or anything else. To judge this would be an injustice to the judged. This authors goal is to help "Turn up the/your 'Light' a little brighter." Not that it's dim. Thank you for your understanding.

Some people say after a two-hour session: "Well, that was a nice massage." Meaning: "No big deal." They call the next day and say: "For the first time in two years I was able to sleep through the night without my leg pain keeping me awake." The process looks and feels simple, and it "cuts to the source" on the pain. One just needs to do the process on a lot of people and see the results. Every session and every person is different. Every result is different in a good way.

The Pyramiding Growth of Pain Over Time

Balancing early pain has the domino effect of resolving later pain. Then your pain in the present has no battery or engine to keep it going. Our process targets and resolves early childhood pain. By removing the earliest pain, present pain is remedied. Inviting your tribe to be a part of your healing helps to heal them and is a benefit to your own healing.

When early pain is removed nerve and immune channels open up and real and long lasting healing can take place. The process in this book blasts the base of this pyramid of pain to pieces. When the base – the foundation of the pyramid that is the source and engine of the current pain – is gone the pain is gone. The present pain one might be experiencing only gets its strength and power from earlier pain. By resolving that earlier pain, the present pain has no battery or engine to keep it going. This is new research.

When a person's early childhood painful traumas and dramas are balanced and realigned, so that they cannot influence decisions in the present life, then life shifts and changes for the better.
Never underestimate the power of understanding how pain works in the body. One can choose to do miracles and choose to be miracles.

The Six Hottest Spots on the Body
An Historic Breakthrough in Healing Research

When we study pressure points and meridians on the body the subject becomes complex very rapidly. I searched for thirty years for the keys to make the subject of healing body energy easy for anyone to learn, to understand, and then to teach.

My research finally paid off. These keys are here given for your understanding and healing now. Focusing on these "Six Hot Spots" gets the fastest and best reliable results.

This concept of body "hot spots" is new. The Heart to Healing Method uses this idea of working with the hottest spots on the body.

The discovery of these six hot spots is revolutionary.

This knowledge was a gift from the Universe, because, with these keys, anyone can follow the steps of a simple process to resolve chronic pain in loved ones.

The six hot spots consist of three on the front of the body, and three on the back of the body:

The Three Hot Spots on the
Front of the Body

(Please see the pictures on the next pages.)

1.   **The Forehead, all of it.**
2.   **The Heart area, front of the body,** and,
3.   **The Don Tien** (Two inches below the belly button and two inches above the pubic bone).

You can practice placing their hands on these three positions on these drawings on the next two pages.
This is a good training tool before working on your partner.

We are spiritual beings.

The spirit needs healing, too.

The Four Healing Quadrants are the

Four Keys Necessary for Healing to be

Complete. Please see the next page.

This Complete Healing System is a gift,

It is for your understanding and use.

Happy Healing!

The Three Hot Spots on the Front of the Body

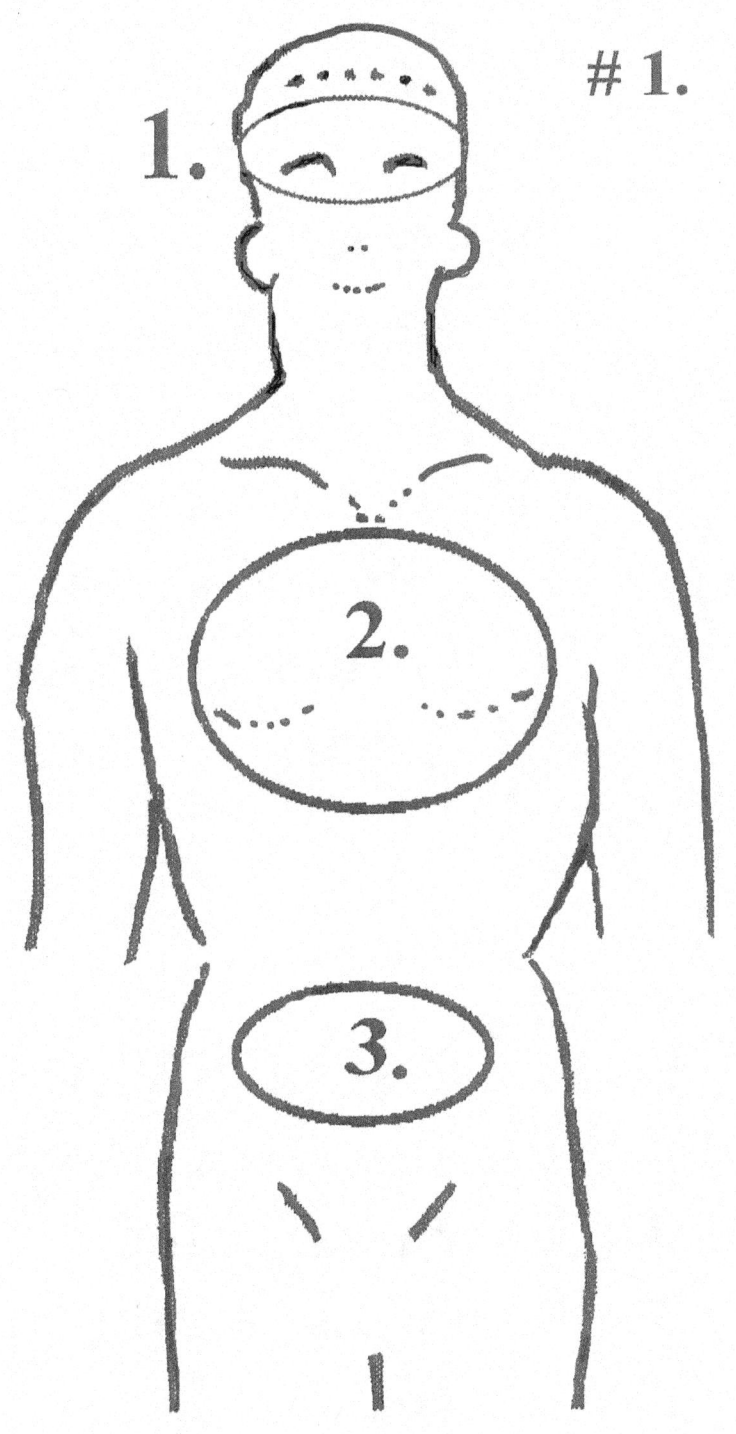

 # 1. FOREHEAD - especially between the eyebrows, and up to the hair line.

2. HEART Area. Front.

3. Don-Tien - 2" below the belly button, & 2" above the pubic bone.

The Three Hot Spots on the Back of the Body

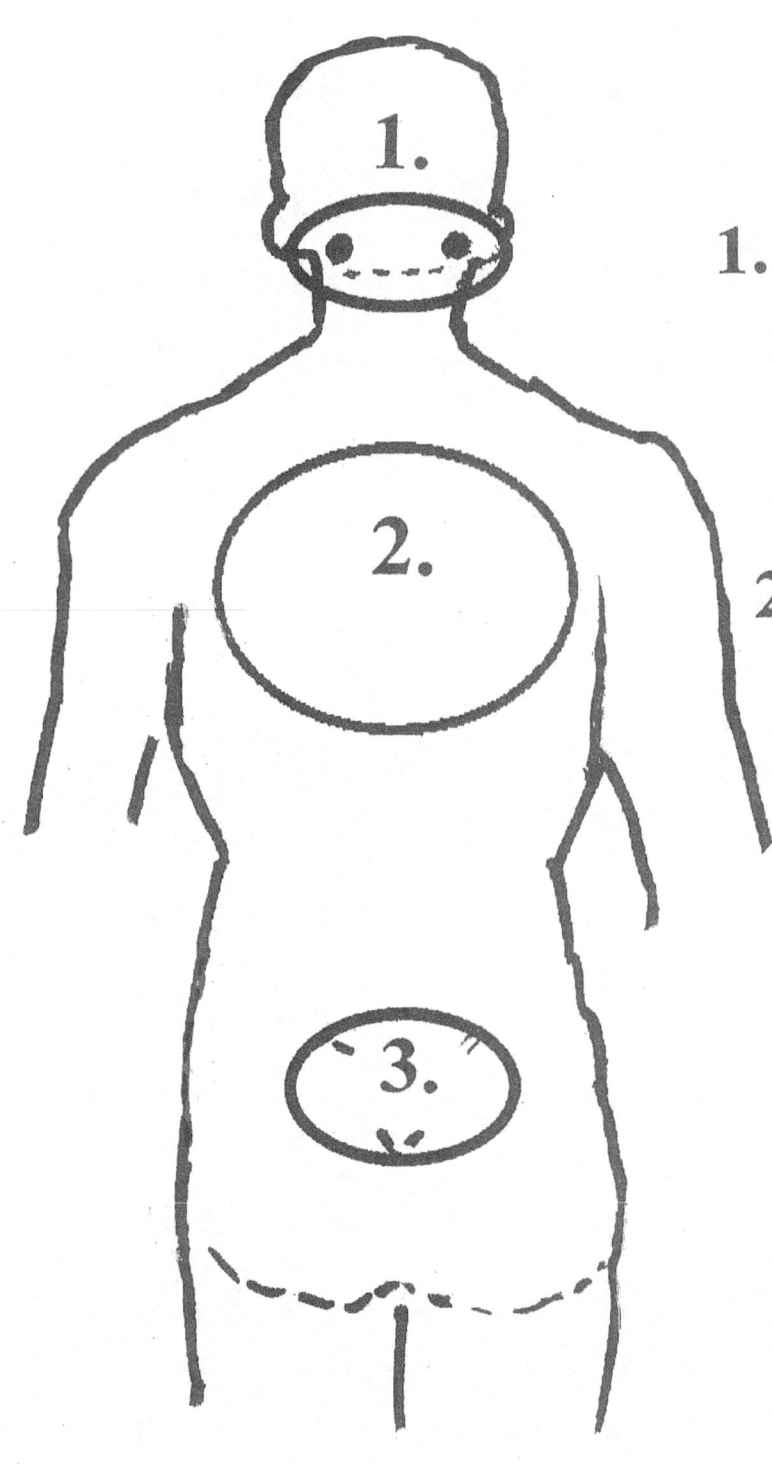

1. **OCCIPITALS** Both. At the base of each ear lobe.

2. **HEART, the whole Heart area.**

3. **SACRUM,** the large hard bone at the base of the spine, at the pelvis.

The Amazing Success of this Healing Method

In September of 2008, I was working on a friend named Mary. She was 80 years old and she had been to scores of doctors and healers in her long life. I had been working on her weekly for six months. She had severe pain in her feet when she walked.

During one session I noticed that there was a ball of energy in her chest that wasn't moving. It had been there a long time. Out of sheer frustration I asked her angels, "What do I need to do to get this stuck energy to move?"

Note: Yes! It _is_ okay for you to ask angels for their help in any healing.

Her angels said, "Put one hand on her sacrum and the other hand on her occipital and let the energy drain."

I remembered that was what the shaman had said to do, so I put one hand on her sacrum and the other hand on her occipital. Shock! Shock! There was a spark at her occipital!
I had been working on her for twenty minutes and I know that it takes a lot of energy to make a spark, so I asked her angels, "What was _that_?" And, "Where did that spark come from?"

The answer came back, "That is traumatic cell energy from long ago, when she was a child."

I knew that Mary had been to many healers for years, so I asked, "Do you mean to tell me that no one ever even got close to balancing that energy?"

The answer came back, "They never even got close."

When Mary got up from the table, I did not recognize her. Her face had lost ten years of age. I asked her to go take a look at her face in the mirror. When she came back she said, "I remember this is what I looked like when I was young." I was amazed, but I had no idea as to the power of this process.

I saw Mary six months later and her face had not gone back to being twisted from the expression of pain, and old looking. I never suspected that the results could be long lasting.

So I asked my angels, "What do I do with this skill?"

They answered me, "Write a book and make healing and energy balancing easy to understand and easy to do."

They knew that I used to write computer technical manuals, so I am skilled at making complex things easy to understand. This is not just a "nice theory," it works very well. After thousands of hours of testing this in energy balancing method, this book is the result of these healing successes.

Note: I still get sparks off of people a few times a year. A spark shows how much energy can be stuck. I have gotten so much heat off of people that observing students have left the room.

Your ancestors energy is healed because you invited them into your healing session and asked them to resolve their past health issues. Asking ancestors and providing a pathway for their healing is huge for your health. This is because no one in the past helped them resolve past health issues. You are the first and you reap tremendous blessings from them for your help. You are DNA connected to your ancestors, and there is a reciprocal effect to your help. Please do not underestimate the importance of this.

The Meaning of Healing for You

Being sick or having a worsening condition produces incredible stress, uncertainty and cost. You are important. Your loved ones are important. Having yourself and your loved ones healthy is important.

Did you know that you, just as you are, can decide to love and help your friends, family, and the people close to you enough that you can make a difference in their healing? Did you know that there is a way to rapidly learn a system to balance body energy that improves immune function and overall health? This is that system.

The good news is that you can learn to do real healing now, today. This process is not instant, but it is faster than anything else out there.

When one starts to do this process it helps to work on your partner for at least twenty to thirty minutes. Then increase the length of your next session to forty-five minutes. Next session try and go for an hour. My ideal sessions are one and a half hours to two hours. I find that the body opens up between seventy and ninety minutes into the session. Let's say you want to end a session in the next ten minutes, and after five minutes your partners body opens up and "dumps a tremendous amount of energy out." My advice is, Let the energy drain out. You waited this long to hit "Pay Dirt" let the energy drain. Your partner carried that energy a lifetime, it's worth allowing more minutes now to release that trauma.

Get Rid of that Chronic Pain -- Fast!

There is no substitute for a strong, resilient immune system. The body knows how to heal itself. Balancing early trauma opens the healing energy so it can flow. Understanding pain and what gives it energy and power is important to resolving it. If you spend some moments studying the "Pyramid of Pain" chart on page 14 you will note that it is the earliest pain which provides the energy to power later pain.

Key: In this healing system, it is the earliest pain that is discharged first. That is, the base of the "Pyramid of Pain," page 14, is blasted apart first. Once the base of the Pyramid crumbles, the entire structure is destroyed. That saves a huge amount of healing time. This is the fastest way to achieve balance of healing energy in one's body that I have found.

This is not an instant process. Rome was not built in a day. The healing relief one experiences is worth the work even if it takes several hours of work. Think about that! What if that were true? Would it be worth it even if it took ten or twenty hours of work - to undo a lifetime of pain? This healing system is about arriving at a level of care where you are willing to do whatever it takes to make a difference in the health and well being of your loved ones. That is certainly better than doing nothing and watching them get progressively worse.

Prove to Me that this Healing System Works.
This is a kinetic learning and healing technique.

Q. Prove to me that this Healing System works.

A. Great question. The answer is in the "Blooming of the energy" of the partner one is working on. Then the proof is in the balancing and resolving of that energy. Please see the answer to this next question:

Q. What is this "Blooming Energy" you talk about in your books, TV shows, DVD's, CD's & lectures?

A. This discovery of "Blooming Energy" is the greatest and most important healing breakthrough in the 21st Century, bar none. When one first touches a partner's forehead, and heart, or don-tien, the warmth of one of the touched areas rises, almost like a stove just being turned on. The energy comes forth, it "Blooms." The energy wants to release and resolve. A cool forehead, upon first touch becomes warm. This can happen almost instantly or more slowly. The more energy there is to be released, the faster the warmth "Blooms." Practice makes perfect. This is a kinetic learning technique. It involves touch, and actually doing the process. One can feel the energy moving, or often, one feels nothing. It does take practice. Heat and coolness are the proof of the energy. This training shows one what to look and feel for, especially for the novice. As one area blooms, the other area tends to cool down. This bloom is the proof of the two-hands hands-on-healing process, proof of the energy being there, proof that there is a "positive and negative" polarity, and proof that the energy can move to balance. Some people may say, "My hands added heat to my partner's forehead," or, "My hands get so warm (hot) when I do this work."

Nice thought, but, "No." It's your partner's energy rising, blooming. This is a major breakthrough in healing as you can feel the imbalance and can then feel the conflict resolve, and witness the healing. It is these processes which train the healer about this stuck energy, and how it resolves. The teaching is in the doing of the processes and in the experiencing, giving and receiving, of these processes. This book is an invitation for you to experience the reality of real balance, real healing, and real learning about a process that works consistently well, with great predictable results. One can work on a partner and not feel any temperature change, however the partner may say afterwards, "Boy. Your hands are the hottest I have ever experienced." They felt the energy and you did not. This is not a problem, it happens. Note: When energy is very deep in the body it may take ten to twenty minutes for the warmth or coolness to "rise" to the surface. Patience is important here. Fingertips are extremely sensitive to heat and cold, a one degree shift is easily felt. There can be a five degree temperature difference between one Hot Spot and another. This difference can resolve quickly to a balanced position.

Ten to thirty minutes of work can move a lot of energy. What this is saying is that one can feel a five degree temperature drop on a persons forehead, heart or don-tien area in as little as a ten minute time period. This is phenomenal speed in bringing balance. Your partner is not done in that time or in an hour or two, but the balancing process has started and new deeper energy can surface, to be handled later.

What Does a Detox Reaction Feel Like?
(The Proof of the Healing Happening)

After this process is experienced the cells in your body can or might dump out toxins. This is just a fact of cells and healing. When cells are traumatized they hold onto toxins to fill the hole left there by pain. A detox reaction might be profound tiredness for a day or two. It is as if you can't even get out of bed. This is because your body is using 90 to 100% of its energy to heal. You can push past this healing but why would you do that? You waited all your life to reach this healing point. Let the healing happen.
You can get your work, projects, and "stuff" done later or tomorrow. We suggest you get plenty of rest and sleep, take "B" and "C" Complex vitamins, and drink a lot of water to flush the toxins out of your body.

Other detox reactions can also be disorientation, lack of depth perception, nausea, dizziness, having the "runs," uncontrollable crying or grief, etc. Sometimes past pain will surface, it will feel the same as it did originally, and it will dissipate and go away in a day or two. Please be careful when you are driving after sessions and realize that your depth perception may be affected. Leave plenty distance around you and other cars on the road. Take surface streets and drive slower than usual if necessary. Please feel free to call this office if the detox reaction gets too great.

Healing Law; "The greater the release, the greater the energy discharge and the greater the detox reaction." This validates the effectiveness of the work you just did.

The Four Healing Quadrants,

Four Keys Necessary for Healing to be Complete.
We are spiritual beings.
The spirit needs healing, too.

Angels & Ancestors, **Including the Spirit,** **and Your Family**	**A Workable Healing Method**
Grounding **!**	**Forgiveness & Gratitude**

Finally the four keys to complete healing have been discovered. This is a healing breakthrough. Each quadrant represents 25% of the complete composition of healing. This is new information.

Do You Only Want to Heal Only Twenty-Five Percent?

Do you only want to heal only Twenty-Five percent (25%)?

How about Fifty percent (50%)? Is that good enough for you? When all four of these elements are present, real healing can take place. Here's the big value secret: You can implement these four keys today into any and all healing modalities and get better results than you are getting now. Even surgeries, even allopathic, even dentistry, homeopathic, Chinese herbs and acupuncture, chiropractic, Ayurvedic, and energy, etc. healing. The spirit-plus-the-physical does a better job of healing than does all the other methods combined. All healing methods are valid. They all work better when the spirit is included. Energy healers all work on the same energy. It's just how we resolve stuck energy that is different. This is a fast healing method. Doing this method teaches you the method. That makes it different, unique, valuable and useful. All the training one needs is in this book. Then practice with friends builds your confidence and that practice makes it perfect.

Considering You, the Spirit in Your Own Healing

All healing goes better when you and your angels and ancestors are included. It costs nothing to ask and the rewards are worth the asking.

Angels & Ancestors

We heal together as a tribe or group. When your tribe heals - you heal. Your tribe includes your angels, ancestors, family and friends, masters and guides, and past pets.* They may have not had the opportunity to heal that which might have killed them. Don't look now but your DNA is a protein code linking you to your ancestor's health issues. That DNA code has their and your health information in it, including their pain and health issues. You can believe it or not. Your belief system changes nothing because that's how it works. Future medical research will bear this out.

* Past pets were and are healing and comforting guides to you and they are included here. Pets need healing, too, because they have similar nervous systems and traumas.

A Workable Healing Method

I don't know any people that say, "I only want to heal fifty percent, half-way." Every cell in your body responds to spiritual energy, this is because life is connected to spirit. Healing is a spiritual event. When one looks at healing as a physical event, that is like being at the ocean, looking intently at a grain of sand, and not seeing the ocean. Healing must address the spirit. Having a workable healing method is such a blessing. It saves you the trouble of, "not having to re-invent the wheel!" And all you have to do is just learn it and do it. People in the healing arts respect methods that work consistently. This healing system works consistently. Try it and you will see. I tell people, "You need to feel it to believe it." It works that well. This author is very suspect of any healing system that does not consider the spiritual side of healing. You have to love and respect the people in your life enough to want to make a difference in their health. This method may be the only place they can get this health balancing help. And it depends on you and your decisions, care and commitment to this work. Someone else just might not come along and do it. It's up to you. Even the medical arts would benefit from implementing these principles of these healing quadrants in their practices and protocols.

> **For example a surgeon could say; "Before I make this first incision, I am asking this person's angels, guides, masters and ancestors to guide my hand, and to be a part of this healing. It is okay for this tribe to heal together with this person."**
> **Try this and see the results. It is worth the effort.**

Grounding

Grounding is very important to healing. When we lived in primitive tribes we walked barefooted, in contact with the ground. Now we live and work in buildings that are above ground. Unless we walk on damp grass barefooted, or barefooted on the ground, or swim in a pool or in the ocean, we rarely are grounded. A good one quarter of healing is grounding. One can get a grounding strap, as is used in computer work, and wear it daily for staying grounded, and use it especially during healing. Ground is the ultimate balance. A good solid physical ground helps one connect spiritually. Remember that the Buddha sat on the ground and meditated to become enlightened. There is no greater holistic healing than grounding yourself. Even organic nutrition (important) and clean (ecological non polluting – non toxic) living is second to grounding.

Forgiveness & Gratitude

Forgiveness has gotten a bad rap in the past. People may hate the concept of forgiveness because it is misunderstood. Forgiveness and gratitude are so high on the scale that it is an injustice and poverty that there is not more awareness and teaching of these principals.

One can do all of the above healing steps except for forgiveness. This limits your healing. My years of working this method with people has shown the failure or unwillingness to forgive holds people's pain in place. Why would one deliberately clip their healing wings by 25%? Again you are responsible for your own health.

On forgiveness one does what one can, realizing that it may take time to completely forgive. One can face a mirror daily and say, "I forgive myself and others that have wronged me." You may or may not believe it. Belief doesn't matter. Just do it. Over time it will become easier to forgive. The phrase, "Forgive and forget" might be better expressed, "Forgive, and learn from the past, and be careful in the future." Part of forgiveness is apology for your wrongs and asking for your own forgiveness. Also, it is okay to continuously thank your angels and ancestors, and the Universe, for their aid, healing and comfort. They do a lot for you without bragging, without show nor fanfare. Thank them, it's okay to show appreciation.

Ancient Healing with a Renewed Twist

During my research, I discovered and revived the ancient custom of hands-on healing. I've brought it into the 21st century. What is new is that it is easy to learn and easy to do. This method of healing is related to Reiki, Acupuncture, Acupressure, Qui-gong, T'ai-Chi, Yoga, Polarity Therapy, Body Talk, Cranio-sacral Healing, the chakras, and all other modes of healing. When this energy balancing technique is used with allopathic medicine it brings the subject into the holistic world of healing. All healing methods should compliment each other. This process works today as well as it did 2,000 years ago. This newness is that it has been studied and refined to be easy to teach and duplicate. Because of the reciprocal healing effect, the gains go quantum distances beyond the actual technique, and beyond the time spent doing the process.

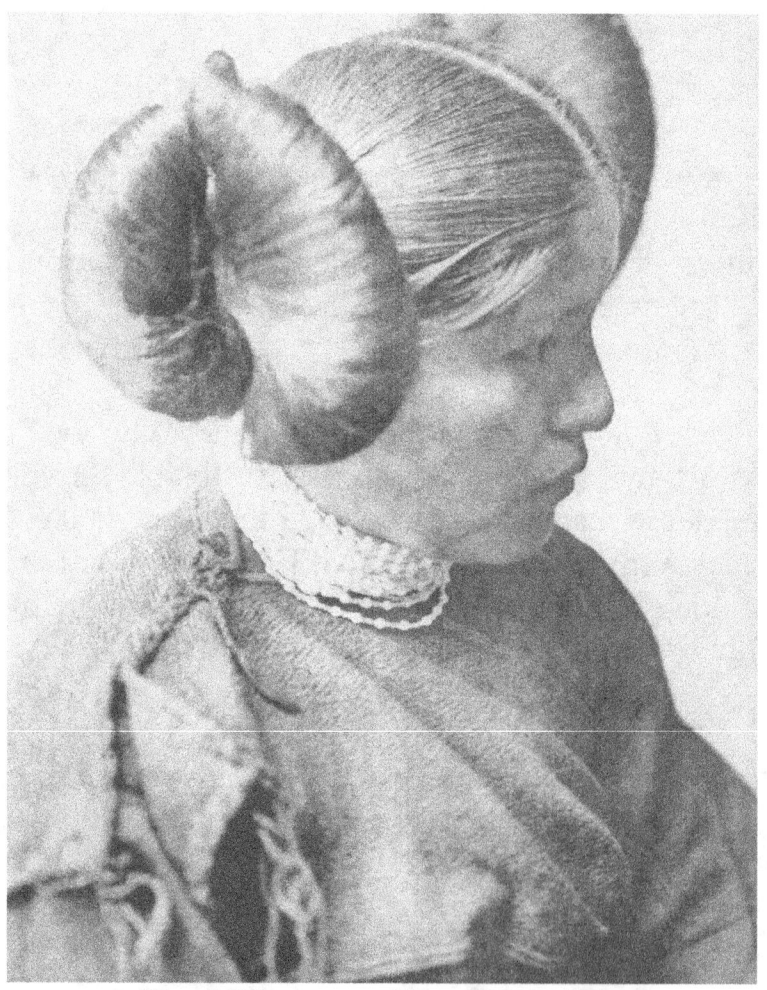

A Hopi Woman – Beautiful Hair

This author is searching for the
Hundreth Monkey (energetically),
and He needs your help by having
You Start and Run Healing Groups
In Your Community!
Especially doing the Global Healing
Parties and Events.

The Story of the 100ᵗʰ Monkey

A story about social change. By Ken Keyes Jr.

The Japanese monkey, Macaca Fuscata, had been observed in the wild for a period of over 30 years.

In 1952, on the island of Koshima, scientists were providing monkeys with sweet potatoes dropped in the sand. The monkey liked the taste of the raw sweet potatoes, but they found the dirt unpleasant.

An 18-month-old female named Imo found she could solve the problem by washing the potatoes in a nearby stream. She taught this trick to her mother. Her playmates also learned this new way and they taught their mothers too.

This cultural innovation was gradually picked up by various monkeys before the eyes of the scientists. Between 1952 and 1958 all the young monkeys learned to wash the sandy sweet potatoes to make them more palatable. Only the adults who imitated their children learned this social improvement. Other adults kept eating the dirty sweet potatoes.

Then something startling took place. In the autumn of 1958, a certain number of Koshima monkeys were washing sweet potatoes -- the exact number is not known. Let us suppose that when the sun rose one morning there were 99 monkeys on Koshima Island who had learned to wash their sweet potatoes. Let's further suppose that later that morning, the hundredth monkey learned to wash potatoes.

Then It Happened!

By that evening almost everyone in the tribe was washing sweet potatoes before eating them. The added energy of this hundredth monkey somehow created an ideological breakthrough!

But notice: A most surprising thing observed by these scientists was that the habit of washing sweet potatoes then jumped over the sea... Colonies of monkeys on other islands and the mainland troop of monkeys at Takasakiyama began washing their sweet potatoes.

Thus, when a certain critical number achieves an awareness, this new awareness may be communicated from mind to mind.

Although the exact number may vary, this Hundredth Monkey Phenomenon means that when only a limited number of people know of a new way, it may remain the conscious property of these people.

But there is a point at which if only one more person tunes-in to a new awareness, a field is strengthened so that this awareness is picked up by almost everyone!

From the book "The Hundredth Monkey" by Ken Keyes, Jr. The book is not copyrighted and the material may be reproduced in whole or in part.

Read the whole book. Healing Authors' Notes:
http://www.wowzone.com/monkey.htm
The 100th Monkey Theory has been on the "Wowzone" site since 1996, and we occasionally receive letters claiming that it was a hoax.

We contacted Penny Gillespie, who was married to Ken Keyes and participated in his work and writing. Here is her response:

The Hundredth Monkey is a real book and hundreds of thousands of copies were printed and circulated, often through university courses. People bought them by the case and gave them away.

The story of the hundredth monkey came from a writing by Rupert Sheldrake. After our book was printed, there was some question about whether the study was authentic. Ken presented the story as a legend, or phenomenon: the concepts of morphogenetic fields and critical mass are very true and the story serves to illustrate them. I hope that answers your question.

All the best,
Penny Gillespie
President's Club, Platinum Wellness Consultant
www.5Pillars.com/pennygillespie

Introducing The Expanded Heart to Heart Healing Process

In the beginning of this book I introduced the basic Heart to Heart Healing Method. One hand on the front heart and one hand on the back heart. Now we introduce the Expanded Heart to Heart Healing Process. With this system, when there is a pain in the back, arm, foot or head, that area is not directly worked on. The areas of the most stuck energy, the 1 – 2 – 3 areas, also known as the "Hottest Spots" are worked on and the pain in the head, the feet, or the back goes away because the source of the pain is gone. (Please refer to the body charts on pages 21 and 22.)

Key: The earliest layer of pain is the layer that breaks up first. That is because this is the hottest, most unstable energy. This is a blessing for the pain sufferer because it shortens the time for this process to work. This makes healing (balance) much easier to achieve.

Earlier pain is the engine that fuels later pain. The present pain one might be experiencing only gets its strength and power from earlier pain, thereby causing a "Pyramid of Pain." So it follows that resolving early pain handles later pain. Thus the present pain has no battery or engine to keep it going. Our process targets and resolves early childhood pain, and by removing the earliest pain, any present pain is remedied. This is huge, as decisions based on avoiding pain from early childhood can crash and burn an entire adult life, keeping satisfaction, employment, relationships, happiness and joy out of reach.

When early pain is removed, stuck channels open up and real healing can take place. The process in this book blasts the base of this pyramid of pain to pieces. When the base, source, and engine of the pain is gone the pain is gone. There is no way to put the pain back except for accidents causing great pain.

The present pain one might be experiencing only gets its strength and power from earlier pain. By resolving that earlier pain, the present pain has no battery or driving engine to keep it going.

The Heart to Heart Healing Method demystifies the subject of healing. This is hands-on healing. This book is for all people to read and be able to use the method the same day. Fast implementation is good.

38

This method consists of a simple process of placing two open hands on another's body, on key hot spots, and waiting patiently for stuck energy to surface and move to a position of balance. It is just like connecting a wire to two poles on a battery to completely discharge it. One is discharging past stuck random trauma energy. Patience and persistence are the keys. You need to care enough about the people in your life to want to make a positive difference in their health.

The good news is that this process cannot be overdone and cannot produce any harm. It has been deliberately made an easy to learn and understand technique. Just trust the process and do it, exactly the same way, waiting for the heat to balance between your hands, showing you that the energy "ball" (stuck energy) has been broken and energy can now flow.

Your sensitivity to this energy and its produced heat – as well as your competence in working with it -- will develop with practice.

The intention is to completely heal people quickly. If you can count to three – "One, Two, Three." – you can learn to heal your family and friends by following this simple process. We all heal together as a whole: The entire tribe of humans and the planet on which we live heal together.

All of this work is at the cellular and spiritual level. It is a waste of time to do it any other way. Sessions are cumulative. This work is long-lasting and does not need to be redone at a later date. The results will be obvious.

Why Don't We Need to Take off the Clothes and Work on the Skin?

This is a blessing to those that feel uncomfortable undressed. There is no need to take off the clothes because some of the energy that you are, as a being, is outside your body. Most people have a one to two inch layer of energy outside their body. Some "sensitives" see this as your aura. It is this energy that the healer is working with. Placing your hands on the clothing makes the best connection. For people that can not, or do not want to be touched, place your hands an inch or two away from their body and the process still works very well because their energy is within that space. Please be patient as it may take a bit longer to see results. It is okay to work on people

People Who Need Several Blankets to Keep Warm

Some people are often cold and require the heat in the room to be turned up, and may need several blankets to keep warm. This is fine. This healing process works even through several layers of blankets. It is important that the receiving person is comfortable at all times.

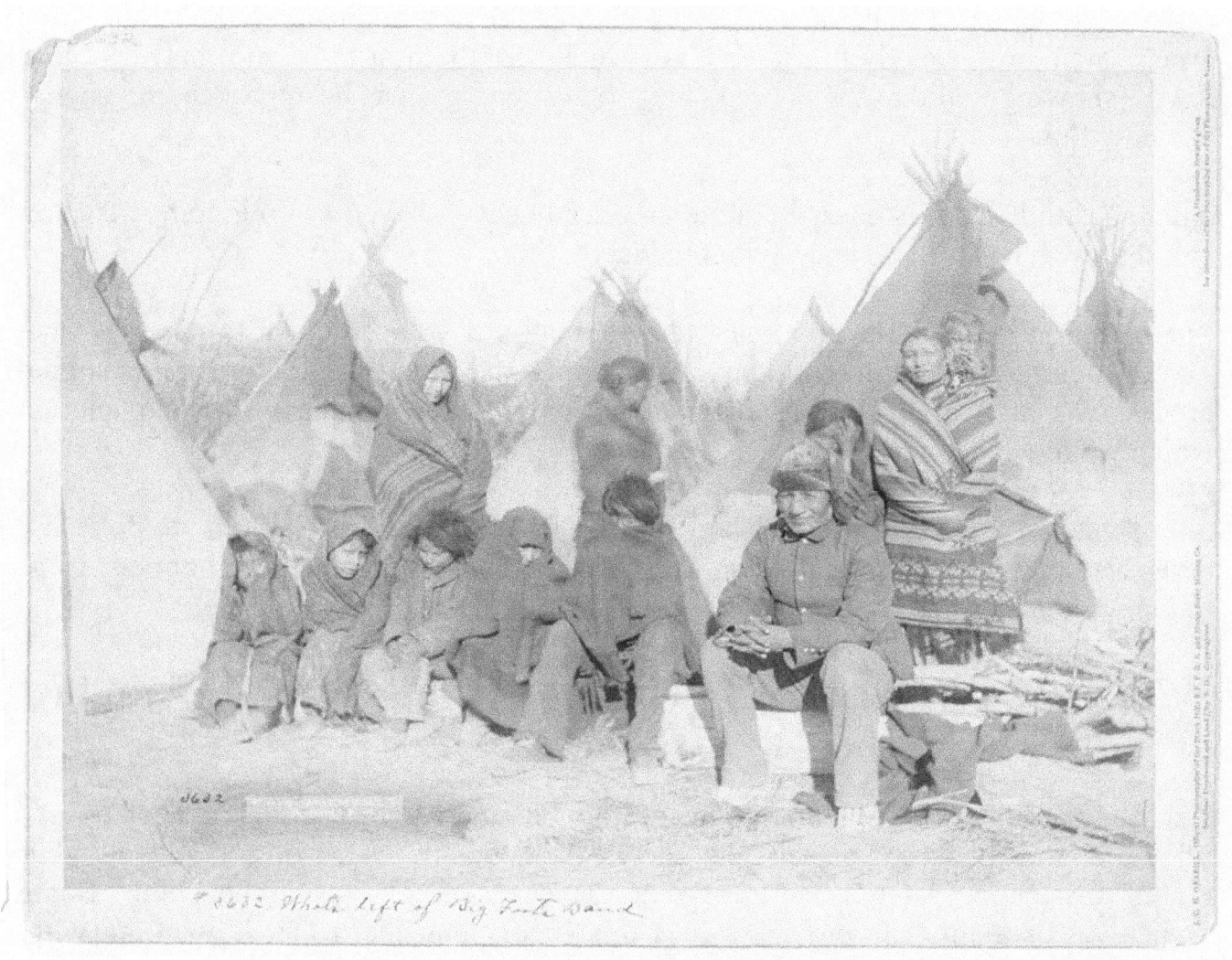

"# 3682 What's Left of the Big Foots Band" 1891

The Expanded Heart to Heart Healing Method

What follows are the exact 1-2-3's of the Heart to Heart Healing "Miracle Worker Process." Do this exactly as it is written – No variations. The best results are received when you follow this by rote. It is important to trust the process until you know from the results that you get that it works well. Just trust the process. As Nike says, "Just do it."

To Begin:

1. Refer to your workmates as "partners" or "friends" to steer clear of legal issues, and always ask for permission to do healing work with and for them. Specifically ask them, "Is it okay with you that I do this healing work on and for you?"

2. Tell them that you will work on the front and back of their body – the forehead, occipitals, front and back heart, belly button, and sacrum. Because you are moving long standing, stuck trauma at the cellular level, the energy starts to move so that real healing can occur. Any mode of healing after that – including homeopathic, aroma, allopathic, nutritional, holistic and manipulative treatments, etc. will be easier, and results will be faster.

3. Have a comfortable place for your partner to lie down. It's nice, but not critical, to have a massage table. A bed, sofa, or even the floor covered with a blanket or sheet with a pillow will work as well. A blanket is okay for cold.

4. Call on your angels, guides and your guides' guides to help in your partner/friend's and your healing. This is done as an application of the "Ask and you will receive" principle.

Guides include angels, ancestors, family, friends, saints, masters, and past pets that have passed or that are still here. Ask all masters, saints, past pets, because they were healing comfort to your partner. People have angels and guides with them all the time. You, and they, are never alone. We all heal together because we all share common energy. This is key. This shifts the view of modern healing. It works because one gets better results when one does it.

You can also call on the great healers of all time to assist with this healing: Saint Michael, the Archangel, Raphael, the Archangel, St. Germane, St. Anthony, St. Francis, St. Theresa of Lisieux, Jesus, the Christ, Mary and Joseph, Emmanuel, King

David, Father Abraham, The Holy Spirit (The Healer), Buddha, Shiva, Confucius, Mohammed, and anyone else you know of. All of your Guides are present with your healing anyway, so you may as well invite them to help and to be healed together. They are all here with you now because there is no time or space on the other side.

5. Your sincerest prayer should be that all of your partner's physical and spiritual issues will be resolved with this session and that this healing work will never need to be redone, except to check and see if the results "Hold." To keep redoing the same work over on the same energy is a waste of precious time, however, new issues can surface, and they do need to be handled as the layers of energy "peel off."

6. Have your partner lie on his or her stomach with his or her back facing up. Say "Now we begin the healing session," or "Now we start the healing session." When you lay your hands on the body, you are completing an electrical circuit. This is key. Because you are completing this circuit you must always have two hands on the body – always. There is voltage there, and your partner's energy can be way off. If your hands get hot and even feel like they are burning – it's the partner's heat, not yours. Stay with the energy until it's all gone and both touched areas on your partners body areas feel the same heat, vibration, and energy. Your partner may feel nothing, or feel the earth shift under their feet. Just do the process. It is more of a heal (balance) process than a feel process.

It is a disservice to leave some amount or "ball" of unhandled energy at any given location. When you find energy, you stay with it until it resolves and balances. There are times when there is no feeling of any energy moving, however, keep your hands there for at least five minutes more. You may be amazed to see and feel what might show up.

Each area could take up to twenty minutes. The area will get hot, cold, soft, or hard, light or dark. As the energy discharges, it will become cool, even, and/or soft.

Hold your hands in place until you feel (intuitively know) that all the energy is discharged. This can get into the intuitive realm, which is a good place to be in healing. Your commitment is to stay with the energy until it is all gone, no matter how long that takes. Once your hands are on your partner it is okay to probe the Hot Spot to see if one area is warmer or cooler than where you first placed your hands.

When Working on the Back

On the back of the body, the 1 – 2 - 3 "Hot Spots" you will work on are,

- **The Occipitals**
- **The Entire Back Heart Area**
- **The Entire Sacrum**

NOTE: The occipitals consist of the bone that runs across the bottom back (base) of the skull, especially at the back of each ear lobe. The sacrum is the hard bone at the base of the spine, at the pelvis. It is the large bone that connects the spine to the pelvis. It is suggested that one first works on the back because many people have mental or spiritual front body "armor" to protect themselves and keep them "safe." They have less or no armor on their back so it is easier to get to the energy. Back energy is totally different from front energy. Practice makes perfect. By doing the process you will develop the feel.

Have your partner lie on his or her stomach, head facing to one side. Pillows are fine. With one open hand (if possible), touch both occipital points behind each ear – touch both sides of the bone at the base of the skull, at the back of each lower ear lobe, where the ear ends. These are the occipitals, and they contain the nerve endings that go directly to the medulla oblongata, the primitive brain that runs the autonomic nervous system. If the head is too wide, just touch one or the other occipital point at the bottom ear lobe.

Touch the sacrum with the other hand, and hold your hands in that position. The discharge of energy can be tremendous, but stay with it until there is nothing left. It can happen in an instant, or it can take up to twenty minutes per area.

High Future Healing Value

Key: This healing goes forward in time to one's children and their children. This method has high future healing value.

The Longer the Discharge, The Greater the Results. Stay with the Process and See the Results. Your Partner's Face Will Soften as the Pain is Released.

There are huge vagus nerve trunks that pass through the spine and sacrum to all the lower internal systems, digestion, elimination, purification, and reproduction organs. The sacrum bears the weight of the upper body, as does the pelvis and both legs and feet. Move to the next area only when there is no more energy to discharge. It is better to err in the direction of taking too much time with this step. When in doubt, spend ten minutes (or more) on each "circuit."

This step cannot be overdone. This "charge" is longstanding and stuck at the cellular level, and it is important to discharge all of it. I have never worked on the same energy twice. When it's gone it's gone. This is so refreshing nor recharging.

When the energy starts to move, the results are profound. Rapid healing can begin. You, the healer, need to understand the importance of this step. Generations are being healed. You are resolving traumas that have been stuck in your partner for their entire live. In this regard, you are truly a miracle worker. As they heal their DNA heals. This ultimately heals the genetic line, per the works of Dr. Bruce Lipton and Dr. Gregg Braden.

Working on the Front

Have your partner lie on his/her back, face up. Place your open hand on your partner's forehead. Anywhere on the forehead is good. There is no need for heavy pressure – whatever is comfortable for you and for them. All you are doing is completing an electrical circuit just like a jumper cable.

Place your other hand just below the person's belly button, and continue until all the heat, energy, conflict is gone. This can take up to fifteen minutes, or however long it takes.

The charge/energy can surface in either hand. Sometimes it surfaces after a minute or two. It can and does switch locations, and it may also alternate hot or cool, hard or soft, light or dark, positive or negative. This alternating can be seen as deep energies waking up, surfacing, and moving through your "jumper cable" hands to a position of balance. Trauma can be mentally carried from lifetime to lifetime, so it may take time to work out all of this energy.

If you find that the energy is really stuck, it helps to coach your partner to take a few deep breaths, and let go of the stuck energy on the exhale. Also have him or her use visualization on the exhale, by visualizing the energy evaporating out of every cell of the body, like mist or condensation – expiring the old away, to make room for fresh new energy.

Also ask him or her what she or he thinks the energy wants, or if they are ready to let go of some of it. Sometimes, with deep emotional pain, there are layers to be unpacked. Like an onion, peeling off layer by layer, then they melt away. Be patient with this energy. It resolves at it's pace not your "expected" time line. You and your partner are worth the time and worth the work. When one realizes how deep the healing goes, a great respect builds for this method. It is deliberately designed to be accessible and learnable. Just because it looks "simple" or "like nothing" does not mean that it does not run deep. These are the heaviest duty processes I have ever seen, and I have seen hundreds of wonderful processes. They are made simple so that people can and will do them. They have little value if people do not do them. One can think or hope about healing all they want. The stuck energy does not move until one completes the circuit with their hands. That's how it works.

If a body part is so hot that you cannot keep your hand on it, ask the person, "What is going on in your head (belly, sacrum, etc.)?" They will tell you. You then can say, "Can you get out of your head (belly, sacrum, etc.) until we finish this session?" They usually say, "Yes." If they say "No." just continue, realizing it will take longer to balance the stuck energy. Never judge their decisions.

Finishing the Session

When you feel your partner is "done," say to their angels, guides, friends and ancestors, verbatim, "Okay, all angels, guides, masters, family members, friends, ancestors, great healers, past pets, 'etcetera,' it's okay to use this persons body now to resolve your past energy issues. You may not have had an opportunity to do this in the past."

This ancestral/angel energy moves very fast – be ready for it. There will be a calm when everything is done. Say to the angels, "Thank you all for helping with this healing process. Your help is appreciated." Say to your partner "This is the end of our healing session." Help them stand up. Tell them, "You might feel a little shaky or dizzy when first standing up. Take your time and get used to it." Give them a glass of water for hydration. Then say, "You may feel tingling up to a week after this session, as the energies sort themselves out. This is good. Be careful if you are driving right away, as your response time and depth perception may be different."

There is No Wasted Healing

The energy that sorts itself out today never has to be worked on again. This is a healing blessing. The balanced energy "Holds." This is true for this healing method. If you find yourself working on the same energy session to session, you need to switch to a method that completely resolves that stuck energy.

The Role of Intuition in Healing

Intuition is good in all healing. Some healers say "I can't feel anything," or "I need to get more intuition during this process." The good news is that the way to get more intuition on this is, "Just Do It." After you have worked on one to half a dozen people, your intuition will just kick in. Just start the process and keep doing it. Doing the process teaches you the method.

NOTE: You might not understand why this process is called "The Miracle Worker Process." Just work on twelve different people using this exact procedure, taking before and after pictures – and if it still doesn't make sense to you, write to this office and tell us of your experience. To others, the reason for this name will be obvious. The before and after pictures show facial changes that happen during the sessions. This is a learning - teaching tool. The faces will never go back to looking the same when all the stuck energy is balanced. This alone is worth the time it takes to get that result.

In the Case of Heavy and Deliberate Abuse of Long Duration

There are individuals who were deliberately abused over long periods of time. This is a sad truth. The energy in their bodies can be stuck in large "balls" of energy in various areas of their bodies. This stuck energy feels "hard" stuck, unmovable. It does respond to this method. It "feels" like a large ball of tightly tied knots, about the size of a softball or larger. When one encounters such energy, one needs to realize that it is going to take a lot of time, care and work to resolve this trauma. Commit yourself to care for that individual enough to do the work necessary to get the job done, "No matter how long that takes." Remember, you are healing a lifetime and a precious being. You also may be saving a life. You heal as they heal. The benefits can be life

47

changing. There has never been a healing method that can undo the trauma suffered in the past as this method does. This is a blessing and a miracle.

My Health is Important to Me.

I Find a Way.
No Matter What It Takes!

How to Stay Grounded

Grounding restores your energy. Remember that all healing is a grounding process. All healing is cumulative. The ultimate balance is ground. People were designed to be connected to the ground that's why we used to walk barefooted. Here are some different ways to get and stay grounded:

Taking a hot bath in a tub that has a metal-pipe water supply and drain pipes connected to it. The drain pipes go to "ground." Ground is neutral, and it is the dirt, the earth of this planet. Add Epsom salts or table salt to the bath water for a better connection.

Walk around barefooted on semi-damp grass for a half-hour to an hour. Lie on semi-damp grass with your bare feet and hands flat on the grass is a good ground.

Get an anti-static strap from an electronic store, and put it on your wrist. Then run a wire from a cold water pipe to where you are resting. That is ground. Put on the wrist strap, connect it to the ground wire, and rest for a half-hour to an hour. The rest will do you good. You can ground your partner, too.

Run a ground wire to the water in your Jacuzzi, and soak in your Jacuzzi for a half-hour to an hour. You may have to turn the heat down so you can stand that amount of soaking time.

Prepare a bowl of warm or cold water with a teaspoon full of Epsom salts dissolved in it, and place both your hands in this solution for half a minute several times a day. This helps ground you. Meditating a half-hour per day, sitting on the ground is grounding, also.

All healing is a grounding process. All healing is cumulative. If one is really concerned with bad energy jumping onto them, they can get two (2) grounding straps from an electronic supply store and connect one strap to themselves and one strap to their partner, before doing this process, and then run both grounding straps to a cold water pipe or to another grounding source. Please follow the instructions that come with the grounding straps. And then do the healing process. It is very important to do the process no matter what. We heal together as a group. Trust this process and do it. The healing one experiences goes way beyond the simplicity of the process. Lives, bodies and generations are being healed.

Note: If you have an indoor cat and it gets outside, the first thing it does when it gets out is to roll around on the ground. The cat wants to get and be grounded.

The Core Principals of this Healing Method

1.   All trauma to the body is recorded and stored at the cellular level. The cells "remember" this pain to keep you "safe" in the future. There is a huge amount of cellular memory. For some reason there is a lot of stored memory of pain in the heart. This is why I developed the Heart to Heart healing method.

2.   There is no "Clear," "Delete" nor "Reset" button to clear this cellular memory.

3.   According to several medical studies, these cellular memories -- if not cleared or balanced -- can manifest as chronic disease later on in life. Please see the "ACE Study."

4.   Dr. John Sarno of Harvard Medical School claims that, "When this early childhood cellular memory is balanced, or cleared, the chronic disease will go away."

5.   Dr. Bruce Lipton made similar statements in his book: *The Biology of Belief.* He stated that you can reprogram your DNA from illness to health.

6.   This is truly miraculous, because nothing like this has ever existed on Earth before now.

7.   Present medical research continues to verify these statements.

8.   After years of exhaustive research, I believe that this "Heart to Heart Healing" method is the only workable method to date that resolves cellular memory of early trauma. And it is relatively fast as a method.

9.   Some people die "natural deaths" much earlier than their normal life expectancy. This book may help to explain why. The longevity implications of this are huge.

10.   The best defense against disease is a strong resilient immune system. One can do things to strengthen one's immune system. We sincerely believe that one can "illness proof" their bodies by having strong immune systems.

Axioms of Healing

With understanding comes responsible control. These principals rule everything you do as a healer:

Energy healing is a service to the Light. Laying on of the hands is a service to the Light. Your intention to help heal someone is sacred. Healing work always goes both ways. You get healed as you heal others. This is worth doing. This is worth the results you get.

Energy Healing is defined as handling the stuck standing energy waves in a body to a point that there is no more static energy to handle. When the static charge – cellular memories/pictures of trauma – are gone, the body's natural energy (Chi) can flow. The body's immune system can click "on" and make future healing much easier. It is impossible to place both your hands on a person without some energy moving in both the giver and receiver. Holding children has a balancing and healing effect.

Do no harm to your partners. They trust you – don't do anything to violate that trust. Always ask your partner if it is okay to work on them. This goes for children, too.

A well-grounded reverence for your gifts, skills, and willingness to help is a big plus. Your work and skill is sacred. You are making a difference to those you work on, to their families, to their tribes and to all of the people of earth.
Welcome any and all guides, angels, and ancestors that show up at any healing sessions.. All are welcome and all need the healing. No discrimination. If you discriminate you limit your own healing.
When you feel tired, take a break and continue later.

Never underestimate the power of teaching the Heart to Heart Healing method to your friends.

This is a powerful, energy-moving technique. There is nothing subtle about it. This technique is similar to Polarity Therapy, with the addition of working with and healing the angels, guides, and ancestors. Generational healing has a multiplier effect toward healing. This system is many times less complex than Polarity Therapy.

In cases of great trauma, like car or airplane accidents, fire, chemical burns, war injuries, PTSD, shock, sexual or emotional abuse, or many surgeries over great periods of time, it may take twenty or more hours of energy work. Here again, patience is the key. Just do the process, and allow the results to flow. The body will eventually release the early trauma.

Remember that the people in your life are worth your care, your attention, your time and your interest in healing them. There is no greater care than taking responsibility for making their health better. You and your whole family win together. In western society it is sometimes easy to ignore or discount the importance of the people in your family or in your life. The message here is that those people are in your life for a reason. Heal them and you heal yourself.

You, the healer, are totally responsible for creating a calm, relaxing, safe, and healing space for your partners. Keep noise and distractions to a minimum. You and your partners both need to turn off your cell phones. Ask your partners if calm music is a distraction or not. Tell them what the music is, and let them decide.

Healing music can be played softly with the partner's permission. "Chakra Suite" and "Paradigm Shift" by Steve Halpern are good. Native American flute music is also good. Classical music works as well, especially light Mozart.

What More Can I Do to Help My Tribe, My Friends, My Community, and the Earth?

Here are some additional things you can do to help your friends, family, and the earth:

If you feel a sincere desire to help in this "push" to heal the people of Earth, you can help by first gathering up family and friends and doing this healing work on and with them. You can listen to music while doing the healing work. The energy moves no matter what. Secondly, get the DVD of this healing method and watch it with family and friends. Then, start "healing clubs," and set an evening aside a week to do this healing on all people that show up. This is why one needs to train others in this Heart to Heart Healing method. You will soon need help. It will snowball. It is okay to ask for love offerings, donations, or whatever, to cover costs. Cook some simple foods like a pot of rice, or cut up raw veggies, or have a potluck, because people will show up hungry, and the healing works better when their attention is on healing and not on food. Show the DVD to newcomers.

There are meet-up groups online that can help you build a dedicated group surprisingly fast.

Get more copies of this book and DVDs, and get your friends to read and watch them. Keep doing the above until you feel the "shift" in global consciousness. You will hear news stories that major and minor diseases are declining on a national or global scale. Please call (408) 253-6577 when you feel this shift. We may be so busy that we don't notice.

Volunteer to help at our events. All are welcome.

Stay connected to the Light, and work toward healing all that need it. Get into nursing homes and hospitals to do this work. There is a tremendous need for things that relieve suffering and improve lives.

Call my office if you ever feel "stuck" (408) 253-6577. This is a healing help desk. Feel free to call us any time for any reason. We are here to help.

What More Can I Do Help Your Organization?

We can use volunteer help with social media, managing our email lists, donations of any sort, phone support when we have an event, people needed to write news and magazine articles. We can use graphic designers. We need branding, advertising and blogging help. We always need writers and editors for articles and books. We need office help. We can use volunteers to learn and take this healing method to churches, social groups, family gatherings, and sports events. We need healers that can invite their tribes to be a part of their healing so as to speed up healing on earth.

Dream with me: Can you picture a world where we are all on an upward healing spiral? Then, as medical science moves forward, we as a people would also experience better health. What about other techniques that are simple and produce profound healing results? There are the advanced healing techniques.

How to Learn this Healing Method Fast

When you experience this energy healing for yourself, giving and receiving, you'll know it works. Teaching this process also accelerates your learning. I believe in total immersion for rapid learning. This method teaches you by your doing the process.

There is a "feeling" to the process. Once you get the feeling, it's like riding a bike, you never lose the skill. Get this book and read it several times. Get several videos from youtube.com and study them, please see page xxxi. Then have a pot luck and invite a dozen friends and have all of them bring something. People will show up for the healing and for the food. Show some of the videos. Then have everyone grab a partner and have them do the Heart to Heart Healing method on each other for ten minutes each person, see page xxii. Use a timer for accurate times. Have people share their experiences. This is a valuable learning tool.

Key: Everyone who shows up gets worked on, even if it's only fifteen minutes or a half an hour each. Everyone doing the process experiences healing because it's a tribal healing experience. This is a great learning tool, have the participants switch partners after each round because they can feel that everyone's energy is different, and it resolves differently. Viva la difference!

Remind the group that the healing work they do is reciprocal, it comes back to them. This is great news for those that have a lot of issues to work through. This is also huge healing energy for their tribes. Please emphasize that more than one person is being healed every step of the way. The stated goal for the group can be, "We all get better together." Get people to commit to return next week for another pot luck and learning session. Have them bring food and friends. Show the newcomers the videos. Then practice the Heart to Heart Healing process. It is okay to have two or more people working on one person. Please be sure to invite all the participants' angels, ancestors, masters, families and guides to be a part of this healing. This greatly multiplies the healing experience. The returning participants can do either the first or the expanded process, pages 52 on.

The trainer oversees the training, keeps the participants in the process, answers questions, and checks occasionally to make sure the energy is moving nicely, and that all the process is complete. You can Call our office if you run into a question you can't answer. You can always ask your angels for their advice. I get instant answers, it has taken some time to achieve that.

People with short attention spans may get bored quickly when they don't see "instant results." Those things in life that are worthwhile take time. Gently train them to meditate or do other things with their mind while the process works. Soft music (or even a TV with tame shows like "Nature") on as background or as white noise as a distraction helps those with short attention spans to maintain the focus necessary. Remind them that Rome was not built in a day.

Entities

Entities do exist. They are beings or energies that "stick" to ones body or to the spirit that is you. Most are neutral, but some are programmed to do damage and harm depending on your past enemies. People from Asia or the South Pacific Islands sometimes have entities. They are cleaned by telling them that they are not needed and to please leave. You treat them as if they are a person standing in front of you and you talk out loud to them just like anyone else. Vocalizing is better than doing it silently. You can ask them for a sign when they leave, or you can ask them to say "Goodbye" as they leave, or you can say "Goodbye" to encourage them to leave. Persistence gets results. In the case of actual possession, it helps to get five healers that understand the severity of the situation to work on the person all at the same time. Set a time to work on the entities and have all five healers work on them and repeat as needed.

Note on Energy: We human beings do share energy. This sharing, or exchange of, energy, occurs especially with people we allow into our own space. We choose our mates and friends based on having or sharing similar energy levels. The magic of this process is that one person gets a healing session and all the people who share energy with them have a totally beneficial energy shift along with them. This is wonderful news. This speeds up the healing process significantly. Healing ones communities is now possible for the first time. Ghosts are handled by asking them what year it is. Do not be surprised if they answer 1853. Tell them today's date and that they were stuck for many years, and that it is okay to get another body or go into the light, or do whatever they wish as long as they leave.

Proof of the Scientific Method
And this Workable Healing Method

This healing method is about you being a whole person.

The scientific method is a set of procedures to establish validity for a study. Part of the scientific method states for a method to be valid, it must be able to be duplicated in any lab anywhere in the world.

This is true for this healing method. It works as well in China, Russia, Africa, all of Europe, North and South America, all of Asia, as well as in Australia and all other countries. This is because people's nervous systems are similar, and cells record pain in similar ways around the world. Try this method in your own country and write to us with your results. To be fair to us, please work on at least twelve people for one hour each before you make any claims as to this methods workability. The reason for working on several people is that everyone is so different and they feel and respond differently.

We remind the readers that Rome was not built in a day. And a person's trauma did not happen overnight. It is so easy to criticize, and so hard to build a healing method that actually works. This process takes time, and work. You and your partner are worth the time and the work. The benefits and the results far outweigh the time and the work for both the giver and the receiver. The proof of the process is in the doing, and in witnessing the results.

When critics foolishly make statements that: "I tried the Heart to Heart Healing Method for five minutes, and it does not work," either they never tried it, or they got it wrong, (there isn't that much one can do wrong!) or they are against anything that might make people and society better. Witness our sad political scene where dis-functionality seems to be what works for them.

That is like saying after drinking/guzzling a pint of Vodka and waiting one minute, "It does not work!" Just wait! What a surprise you are in for!

There is a remedy: Get this book, master the method and give these naysayers a session! Start with the Heart to Heart healing process and work up to the full expanded six-point "Hot Spot" Expanded Heart to Heart healing method.

I am a great admirer of Sir Frederick William Herschel. He discovered infrared light in 1800. What makes him a brilliant scientist is that he designed an experiment that showed that what one cannot see is actually there. Until then all of science was based on: "If I can see it in my own lab than it is real, seeing is believing." And: "If I can't see it than it is not real." Bravo! Scientists that think outside the box.

Scientists of the Future

Scientists of the future will design experiments that show spiritual things that can not be seen are there and are real. What a relief that will be.

How Can I Get More Information on Getting Rid of My Chronic Pain?

Please call (408) 253-6577 now and make an appointment to get a free introductory session. You will need to come to San Jose, California for this as this author rarely travels due to his busy schedule.

Imagine you, with no pain and a body that works surprisingly well and with lots of energy. Call now.

Note: We are raising $250,000.00 (two-hundred-fifty-thousand dollars) to produce a PBS special on getting rid of chronic pain based on this method. This PBS Special will be of the quality of Dr. Deepak Chopra, Dr. Wayne Dyer, etc. We pay a 10% commissions to those that help us raise this money. Please let us know if you know of people who donate to such projects.

What You Can Do, Today to Help Get
This Method Widely Known and Used.

It is important to get this information widely known and used in every part of healing. This technique can speed healing, reduce pain, cut medical costs, and save lives. Tweet it, blog about it, mention it on Facebook, Pintrist, and the other social media channels. One can even write or tweet talk show hosts about this method.

Please, tell your family, friends and medical professionals, even buy bulk copies of this book and hand it out to people who need healing. Please tell everyone you know far and wide. It costs nothing to mention that there is a way to heal and a way to balance the body's energy. If you know people who have TV studios, who produce or host their own TV or radio shows, or anyone who has any sort of advertising channel or media, please tell them that I would love to be invited to their show. Bulk copies of this book are less expensive that buying through bookstores ro through Amazon. Please call our office for prices.

Frequently Asked Questions:

Q. What is my commitment as a healer to my partner?

A. Excellent question. Your role as the healer is to care enough about your partner be they a child, a parent, a friend, etc. to stay with the energy until it is resolved. And to continue working on them over time until all issues are resolved. Practice on a lot of partners teaches one the finer differences between people and the subtlety of the energy one is working with. Your skill sharpens with every session. Your healing is reciprocal. The healing you give comes back to you.

Q. What if I feel nothing, and my partner feels nothing?

A. This is fine. Just keep doing the process. Any chronic pain or chronic condition that lingers shows that there is energy still there to handle. My greatest sessions ever were when I felt nothing and my partner felt nothing for hours.

Q. Are there any people that don't need this process?

A. Yes. They are extremely rare, maybe one in a thousand. A good rule is that if a person ever had a serious fall as a child, or was whipped, or fell from a tree or jungle gym, or hit in the head with a ball in sports, broken a bone, or in a car or other accident, they can benefit from this process.

Q. Is it okay to take breaks?

A. Yes. Take a break whenever you or your partner needs one. Always tell your partner that you are taking a break so they know.

Q. Is this like "Reiki?"

A. Yes. It is like Reiki in that stuck energy is moved and balanced. It is unlike Reiki in that the energy the healer is targeting is the original trauma that fuels/energizes later pain. My Reiki friends tell me that this process is at least two steps "Pre-Reiki." And they use it before their Reiki sessions. They say that it makes the Reiki sessions run faster and smoother, and they get more referrals.

Q. I was working on a good long time friend and her chest felt hard like a barrel. Her chest would not expand or contract like normal when inhaling, nor exhaling. What is that?

A. Your friend may have serious issues going on in her body. Whenever things don't feel normal in a body, have them get to a doctor quickly. Serious illnesses often have no pain and give no warning signs. What works for this author is: I ask her to pick up her cell phone and dial her doctor and make an appointment right then and there. One never diagnoses nor treats anything, but one can help by insisting their friend get to a doctor as soon as possible. This is a critical point. Your friend might have been suspecting something is going on, or they are clueless. It is your job to make sure the appointment is made right then and there. Serious illnesses can often be stabilized with modern medical treatments. Get your friend to a doctor fast, you may be saving a life. If not balanced, the past pain can solidify in the body.

Q. What can I do to help this work progress?

A. One can help by learning and doing the process. Simply schedule some time during the week and take the time to help a friend or family member. Remember, it only takes a commitment of time to do this process and eventually get a result. Secondly, one can volunteer to help our healing organization. Thirdly one can start healing groups or clubs in their area that meet weekly or bi-weekly. Fourthly: One can contact local and national media organizations and ask them to interview this author. There is power in many requests coming into a show or to a station for an author or presenter. Fourthly one can use all the social media they are on to get the word out wide and far.

Q. Do these processes handle past life trauma?

A. Excellent question. Yes. These processes handle all of the trauma and energy that is stuck regardless of the time line. If the energy is stuck, these processes will move it. This is profound, this has not existed on Earth before now. Please let your friends know about this. Tweet, and use Facebook and social media to create "Buzz." This work is important and needs to get out there. Please help this author make it go viral on the Internet.

Q. A friend of mine came to me and said they were terminal with a major fast advancing disease. They asked me to work on them. What should I do?

A. I am sorry to hear about your friend. I have lost several close friends that way. Have them get a doctors note giving them permission to get energy healing. This is important. Often partners come to this author that are terminal, and they say that they don't want to go through this agony again on the chance that they decide to return to Earth. I make sure the energy treatment is okay with their doctor. I make absolutely no promises, and I make sure they know that there are no guarantees of anything. Once they know these ground rules, then I work on them. They are very grateful for the healing work.

Subtle Note: This author does believe in miracles… This author has seen miracles… And this process is a miracle…

Use it for your benefit and for the benefit of others.

Q. Do these processes handle early childhood trauma and abuse like rape, severe punishment and abandonment?

A. "Yes. Yes. And Yes." This is a major key to healing deep intentionally inflicted pain. It may take a lot of hours of work, sometimes 30 to 50 hours, but it is like handing the person a whole new lifetime. All the decisions they may have made about unworthiness, confusion, violation, fear of people, etc. can sort themselves out and they can make decisions in present time based on present information. This is a miracle, and processes like this have not existed on Earth before now. Working on people that were abused "feels" like untying a huge ball of "very tightly tied knots of stuck energy." Few things that one does in life are as rewarding as releasing a person of the "prison of trauma" that early abuse is. After this process is done partners tell this author, "Thank You, Paul, for giving me back my life."

When one tries to figure out, "Why everything I touch turns to crap," the answer may lie in their early trauma, or abuse. Life is different when one balances that early trauma.

Q. What is the purpose of these processes, what is the benefit, and why do I need this?

A. Because pain is cumulative, and because that accumulation can block or shut down nerve and immune flows in the body, and can ultimately manifest as chronic illnesses these processes are used as:

1. Preventive measures, like vitamins and supplements, for increased energy and focus,

2. Handling present and past chronic pain,

3. Bringing balance to stuck energy wherever it occurs,

4. Resets the effects of past trauma to zero!

5. Recovery of lost life force due to pain avoidance,

6. Handling depression, better sleep, easier to meditate and relax,

7. Peace of mind, tranquility, better spiritual connection,

8. Bringing balance to stuck energy opens nerve, blood and immune channels that were previously blocked.

9. The body has wisdom and knows how to heal itself when the blocks to stuck energy are removed.

10. This is a true miracle working process. And this healing method has not existed in this simplified form on Earth before now. Please jump on this opportunity to help yourself, your friends and your tribe.

Q. Why must I always put both my hands on my partner?

A. **Excellent question.** Thanks for asking. Your hands are like a car's jumper cables. You are connecting one "Hot Spot" with another and allowing the accumulated energy between those spots to discharge. The proof of the discharge is the heat or coolness that one feels during the process.

Q. Can I do any harm to my partner with these processes?

A. **No.** If there is no energy that is stuck, then it just feels like a nice massage, and we all can use a nice massage now and again.

Q. Can this process rebuild the cartilage in my knees?

A. This is a basic energy balancing process. It can not replace what is already lost.

Q. Can these processes handle PTSD and depression in returning veterans?

A. "Yes!" PTSD is caused by being in extremely stressful, highly dangerous situations. The stress is so great that it is recorded in the cells as being traumatic.

Q: I was working on my wife and her forehead and heart kept getting warmer and cooler and never got to what you call "balance?" What should I do?

A: You are doing the process right. Alternating warmer and cooler areas show the energy is moving. Keep doing the process, even if it takes many sessions, and it will eventually balance her energy. The heat and cold prove that the energy is there to be balanced. Your work is cumulative, it is not lost when you take a break.

Q: Why would the author spend the time to write another book on healing? Aren't there enough books out there already about healing?

A: This is a brand new subject to launch into the world. Spirituality, angels, ancestors and grounding finally become part of the healing equation. What makes this book so valuable and unique is that this pain elimination system works very well and it makes the subject of energy, pain and healing simple to understand, fast to learn, and easy to do. This is new, this is unique, and this has huge value. This is a healing breakthrough. It's a new science.

Q: Why would one ever want to heal with their ancestors and angels? What a concept."

A: We are moving into a new age of healing. That is what December 2012 was all about. There has been a shift in consciousness. Global spiritual awareness is accelerating. Also, we all heal as a group or as "a tribe." As the tribe energy is healed the members of the tribe heal. This method was only known to a few, now it is released to the public. Look around, this world needs a faster healing method.

Q: Can another person's bad energy or trauma jump off of them and get on me? Or vice-versa? Is there any kind of danger like this in the process?

A: No. that is an excellent question. It was early trauma that caused the partner's energy to get stuck. You, the energy worker, did not have the same trauma. All you are doing is discharging that stuck energy. The energy exists between the "Hot Spots" within the partner's body. The discharge is between the cells between these Hot Spots. Their energy is totally separate from you and yours. Picture a car battery and a set of jumper cables, and one connects one side of the cable to one terminal of the battery, and then touches the same cable to the other terminal of the battery. There is a huge spark and a lot of electrical discharge. How much electrical energy jumps out of the jumper cable and battery onto you? Honestly, none to speak of. And how much energy does the jumper cable absorb? None, really.

It is also recommended that two people partner up and read the book together and do the process on each other in turns. That way any extra energy that builds up is discharged. This sharing of healing works well in small and large groups. The rule is that everyone that shows up gets worked on.

Q. Can this Heart to Heart Healing Process be done during sex with my life partner?

A. **Yes, with great care.** You can't be in a speed contest to see who can finish first. Your intentions are for a sacred healing session during this time together. You go slow, hold your partner, plan on staying connected for at least half an hour. Both of you hold your partner's heart area with both hands, for the whole time. When one does sex as a caring, healing process, loving takes on a whole new meaning. Healing can be fast, powerful and deep. This author wrote a private article several years ago about sex and healing. It is called "The Pelvis Protocol." It is for clearing deep sexual trauma. This study will never be published in book form because it is a private study/paper. Call or email this office for more information on getting this study. Like all this author's writings, this process works very well.

These Principals Guide All Healing of All Modalities

1. This healing system is complimentary to all other healing modalities. It is not medicine, chiropractic practice, nor massage. It does deal with energy and the spiritual world.

2. Permanent healing heals the spirit as well as the body.

3. Effective healing of the body is possible.

4. Healing one's ancestors is possible, and so is healing one's present family members.

5. Ancestor health issues can be resolved in the present because the energy of the illness is still stuck. It is so stuck that it killed them! When it is resolved it will set you free! Your DNA carries the good and stuck energy of your ancestors. You can un-stick the past ancestral energy.

6. Healing your friends' pain is possible, and so is healing your own body/spirit.

7. Remote healing is possible because we are all connected, and we heal as a tribe/group. This is true even if you don't believe it.

8. Healing past life pain and emotion is possible, and happens in these sessions.

9. Asking for and including ancestors, angels, guides, masters, friends, family members and others to be a part of the healing is beneficial, desirable and possible.

10. No one needs to live with pain with this new healing system.

11. This healing method is cumulative – today's results are not lost tomorrow, even partially balanced energy remains balanced for a long time. And balancing of the body's energy continues even past the session's end. This is unique in the healing field.

12. There is a multiplier effect to doing this healing work. You get or give a session and your family members can get better.

A year ago I worked on a lady here in San Jose, California, who had a mother in Boston, Mass. who was having health issues. She had me work on her for the benefit of her mother. After the session and before this lady got home, her mother called from Boston and said she was doing much better! This is because there is no time nor space in the spiritual realm. Everything is present. Results like this are possible and common.

All of the above is major good news because healing like this has not existed on Earth in an easy to understand, and easy to do system before now!

This needs to be shouted from every rooftop, and tweeted continuously. Please tweet and blog this news for this not-to-tech-savvy author.

Pages 68 through 72 Are A Taste of What's in This Author's *Angelology* **Book. This is in Addition to wonderful information about Angels, Ancestors and spiritual connection.**

Author's Opinion: Dr. Oz, Dr. Mercola, Dr. Amen, Dr. Perricone, Dr. Deepak Chopra, and other alternative medical doctors say that inflammation is the precursor to all major diseases including cancer, stroke, and heart disease. Read "inflammation is the precursor to all major diseases." This author has the shocking view (highly unpopular - controversial) that if a person wanted to "prevent" major diseases in their own bodies, that maybe managing inflammation in their own bodies "might" be a way to do that. Especially if one smokes and can't quit, and if one has a family history of members dying at a young age of major diseases. Now how does one do that? How can one tell if they have inflammation? Look in a mirror at your face. Is it "puffy" or soft around your cheeks, or chin or throat? Touch these parts and see if they are puffy or soft. Make a fist, and look at the backs of your hands, feel them and see if they feel puffy or soft. That's inflammation, and it can be managed and controlled. By the way, foods that contribute to inflammation are refined sugar, fructose, dairy, and wheat/gluten products, synthetic cooking oils, and others.

I write these things to get this healing news out to the people. "My people suffer from want of knowledge."

A Note on Smoking

This author believes that smoking creates a perfect environment for inflammation to take hold in your body, and creates a perfect environment for disease. Once one quits smoking your body detoxifies **50%** of the smoke related poisons the first year of quitting. Each additional year your body gets rid of **50%** more of the remaining toxins. Most major cities in the U.S. have **FREE** smoking cessation clinics. Read "**FREE**." They understand that it takes a community to quit. They understand the threat to health that smoking presents. Please Google "**FREE** smoking cessation clinics" in your area for your own good.

There is hope… It takes a village. **Note:** E-cigarettes are a blessing to those trying to break the smoking habit. They are a quitting aid. One uses them to reduce addiction to nicotine and thus the urge to smoke. They gradually help to taper the smoker off of the nicotine. Popular equating of e-cigarettes to smokers enjoying a cleaner addiction do not understand that they are a practical withdrawal tool. Thank goodness there is relief from smoking.

Note: Please do not abuse e-cigarettes as a lesser evil to the 1000 poisons in cigarettes. Nicotine is a powerful nerve poison. So is alcohol in all it's forms. There is nothing "fun" nor "social" about powerful nerve poisons. And you are smart enough to figure out an alternative to your stressful life style other than alcohol or nicotine. And if you are not smart enough to figure it out, please ask a professional or a friend as to how to get it done.

Handling Your Bodies Inflammation

Rescue & Strengthen Your Compromised Immune System

A traditional Old World remedy for colds, infections, and inflammation, etc. given to Paul Barbaro by Dr. Ray Evers, M.D. in 1995. Doctor Evers was an early founder of the Holistic Natural Foods movement in the late 1940's and early 50's. The FDA despised him and tried to stop him and his work... I wonder why? He dared to grow his own organic foods and feed organic vegetables to his sick and dying patients. He paid the price for this horrible outrageous medical crime at that time with his life. This formula helps reduce infections, inflammation, and improves immune function, as well as nourishes healthy cells. This drink is not an instant healer. Rome was not built in a day. It takes time to reverse a compromised immune system. If one has a chronic health condition one needs to do this drink every day for at least two months. One gets used to the taste. Here's the recipe, it works miraculously well, especially when nothing else even touches the inflammation:

Bring to a boil 32 ounces of water in a pan on the stove. When boiling shut it off.
While it is heating up dice two medium sized lemons. Take out the seeds because they are bitter. Dice skin, pulp and all and put it in the boiling water. Shut off the heat & steep for six minutes only. The hot water softens up the lemon so it blends easily. Do not use an aluminum nor an iron pan as the acid will react with the metal.
Let it cool for about 10 minutes and put the entire mixture into a blender and blend until it is a smooth puree. Add honey or other sweetener because it is very bitter. You may have to add cool water to thin it down.

Drink eight ounces of this lemon tea every four hours, all day long. The cold, or infection should be gone in a few hours, or overnight at best.

It works because all you are doing is adding huge amounts of Vitamin C and Anti-Oxidants to your body.
The doctor told me the reason to use the pulp is because 98% of the lemon's Complex Bioflavenoids ("C –Complex") are in the pulp. Your body's natural state is healing. When you get cut you naturally heal. All the lemon does is boost the strength of your immune system. Lemon tea is immune support until your body can do it for itself. The fact of sickness, or inflammation is proof of the compromised immune system. Vitamin C, by the way, is an antibiotic and antibacterial. So is garlic. You can't

overdose on Vitamin C or lemon juice because it's a natural food. I have gotten so used to the taste that I no longer boil the lemon nor add sweetener. Optional variations of this recipe: I now add two cloves of garlic, and a 2" to 4" inch ¼ inch wide strip of ginger, (Yes. Chinese style ginger.) and a 2" inch strip of fresh aloe vera (cut off the spines, and don't skin it.) and put them all in the blender with the lemon mixture. Garlic, vitamin C and ginger are anti-bacterial, anti-inflammatory, and anti-microbial, and are antibiotic (kills invading, "bad" bacteria). This is a good thing. I hope this helps. Add half an orange to naturally sweeten this drink.

Did you know that chemo therapy destroys one's immune system? And that the chemo patients have down time after chemo therapy to repair their damaged immune system? Doesn't it seem that one should be trying to strengthen one's immune system when one is sick, rather than to destroy it? A strange thought indeed.

Author's Note, I no longer heat up the lemon drink. Over time I have gotten used to the bitter taste and it no longer bothers me.

An Easy GELATIN Recipe to Handle Joint Pain, and Help Rebuild Lost Cartilage.

(Jell-O = gelatin = cartilage = padding between bones.)

Every bone, joint, ligament, and cell membrane in the body contains cartilage also known as gelatin, the same as "Jell-O." Gelatin is made by boiling animal bones to get the cartilage from them. Whole Foods and Sprouts has a plant based, non-animal gelatin for vegans and vegetarians. Minor joint pains can be remedied by drinking a warm eight ounce gelatin mixture two times a day, for four weeks. This goes for back pain, also, as the spinal disks and knee cushioning are made of this gelatin.

When one drinks gelatin daily it strengthens joints, ligaments, muscles, cell walls, bones, nails and hair. One can not overdose on gelatin/cartilage because it is food and the body will burn it as a fuel when it is not needed to strengthen body parts. A carnivore diet simply can not provide one with enough cartilage to rebuild joint cartilage.

Recipe:

Two quarts of cold water in a three quart pan, while stirring mix in 3 to 4 heaping Tablespoons full of Knox unflavored gelatin, get it at Smart & Final, at Amazon or other online sources. It's about eleven dollars a pound, plus the cost of flavoring and or sweetener. While stirring mix in 3 to 4 heaping Tablespoons full of flavored Jell-O or other flavoring. Optional: Add stevia, honey, xylitol, agave or other sweetener to taste if necessary. Mix all the above cold, it mixes easily cold. Mixed cold, it does not lump. Let it stand 5 minutes to let the crystals dissolve, then, on medium heat, heat the mixture up while stirring continuously. Do not boil, when the mixture goes "clear" in color it is ready to drink. It starts out cloudy and goes clear when luke warm.

Paul Barbaro, the healer, got this recipe in 1995 from a man that did sports injury medicine. He knew his subject. This works. Try it today, Jell-O is an inexpensive fix for
mild annoying joint pain.
(Jell-O is a registered trademark of Kraft Foods).

Success: I have suffered with painful knee joints for over a year. I was taking pain medication daily. This morning I tried Mr. Barbaro's gelatin drink and by the evening I noticed that the pain was quite a bit less by half. I am impressed. Imagine a remedy that costs less than $15.

Rhonda T., San Mateo, California, 2014

Improved Memory and Brain Performance

In this high performance world one needs all the brain and memory power one can get. What works? Please see below.

Students and people in high-brain – memory demanding jobs need to keep sharp for a minimum of eight hours a day. B-Complex multi vitamins really help. One starts with 50 mg and later can progress to 100 mg of a good B-Complex multi vitamin. "Trader Joe's" and "Whole Foods" have decent B-Complex multi vitamins. When extremely high brain function is a must, add Niacin, 50 to 100 mgs to the B-Complex regimen. One can get a "Niacin flush" if one takes too much. This is harmless, but produces a "prickly pin" sensation all over the skin, and one can turn as red as a lobster when the blood vessels in the skin open up. Niacin is good in helping the blood carry oxygen to the brain. The brain runs on oxygen.

Caution: Caffeine triggers Niacin. Be very careful with coffee and caffeinated soft drinks until one knows how one responds to these stimulants. By the way B-Complex and Niacin is a better way to "click the brain on" than caffeine or energy drinks. This is because caffeine and energy drinks burn up reserve vitamins and energy in the body, and one crashes due to the lack of nutrition in one's body.

Do not take Niacin nor B-Complex after 2:00 PM because it will be hard to get to sleep at night. If one can not get to sleep, melatonin and L-ornithine counteract the sleepless and "over active brain" effect.

Some Acknowledgments:

We are deeply thankful to Deepak Chopra, M.D., Joseph Mercola, M.D., Joseph Maroon, M.D., Dr. Joel Fuhrman, Dr. Lisa Rankin, Dr. Bruce Lipton, Dr. Gregg Braden, Alex Loyd, M.D., John Sarno, M.D., Ray Evers, M.D., Laura Day, M.D., (she beat cancer), Mehmet Oz, M.D., Dr. Michael Roisen, M.D., Carolyn Myss, Louise Hay, the United States Army, George Carr, MD, Carl Ferreri, M.D., Dr. Mitchell Corwin, and hundreds of other alternative treatment doctors for their ground breaking research on nutrition, methods that work and on cellular memory as the original source of pain.

Special thanks is given to Dr. Wayne Dyer, Ram Dass, John Gray, Ronald Downey, Sri Bhagavan and Sri Amma, and hundreds of others, for their continuous pioneering of new ways to chart spiritual and healing discoveries. Special thanks also to Joseph Campbell and my parents and tribe.

Reference Materials

Dr. Mehmet Oz, http://www.doctoroz.com/

Dr. Joseph Mercola, www.NaturalNews.com

David Wilcock, http://video.google.com/videoplay?docid=-4951448613711060908&hl=en

Divine Cosmos, http://www.divinecosmos.com/index.php?option= com_content&task=view&id=12 (David Wilcox's site)

http://www.tryitoneverything.com/ (EFT)

http://www.oprah.com/article/oprahandfriends/moz/20080916_oaf_moz

http://www.curezone.com/cleanse/liver/

http://www.curezone.com/schulze/herbal_5day_liver_cleanse.html

http://www.puristat.com/livercleansing/livercleansingdiet.aspx

http://www.thejourney.com

Suggested Reading

Any Books, CD's, DVD's by:
- **Dr. Mehmet Oz, M.D., www.doctoroz.com/**
- **Dr. Barry Sears, M.D.,**
- **Dr. Deepak Chopra, M.D.,**
- **Dr. C. Everett Koop, M.D.,**
- **Dr. Daniel Amen, M.D.,**
- **Dr. Joel Fuhrman, M.D.,**
- **Dr. Andrew Weil, M.D., www.drweil.com/**
- **Gregg Braden**
- **Carolyn Myss www.myss.com**
- **Carol Sutherland**
- **David Wilcock http://divinecosmos.com**
- **David Wolf**
- **Nick Delgado**
- **Wayne Dyer**
- **Paul Barbaro www.healingangelguides.com**

- Bruce Lipton
- John Gray
- Michael Bernard Beckwith, Agape Center of Truth
- Jacqueline
- Marianne Williamson
- Dr. Carl Ferreri, D.C.,
- David Wolf
- Hay House
- Sounds True, et al
- Dr. Mark Hymen, M.D.,
- Dr. Steven Masley, M.D.,
- Dr. Robert H. Lustig, M.D.,
- And hundreds of others whose input was a tremendous help. Viva la research that discovers healing methods that actually work.

So What? I am a Surgeon, What Good is this Healing Method?

Great question! When you are all suited and scrubbed up, and the patient has been prepped, and you are ready to make the first cut, you say out loud, "I ask my angels and your angels, and I ask my and your ancestors and family members to be a part of this healing, and to guide my hand during this surgery." And then you make the first cut. By saying this the entire Universe lined up to support you, and that made all the difference in the world. Try this and see if recovery times improve. Try this and see if the law suits go away.

Tell me More About Your Books

"Angelology" is your next book because it has tips for staying healthy. How to strengthen your compromised immune system, How to re-colonize your gut when antibiotics kill off the good bacteria, and a lot more tips on staying healthy. This book is a wealth of information about making a better connection with angels, ancestors, guides, saints, and the spiritual realm. **ISBN - 13: 978-1496132178**

"Healing Our Community" – This is a rapid, powerful group healing process. Hundreds can be healed in minutes. It can be used for healing from three to one-thousand people. The process runs for about fifteen minutes in a circled group setting. This provides real healing for our communities and for our nation.
ISBN - 13: 978-1495281457

A Word to My Critics!

One earns irrelevance by their criticism. The path to invisibility is criticism. There has never been a statue erected to a critic. You have the power to arrive at your own observations and conclusions without the opinions nor criticisms of others. Take this opportunity to arrive at your own conclusions. I don't want you to believe anything I say! I am not your opinion leader. Please avoid people who are more critical than they are positive.

I once had a prominent medical doctor ask me, "How can I make a lot of money doing your healing method. I told him that besides charging by the hour, this method does not help sell a lot of drugs nor surgeries. I told him that he doesn't need this method until there is someone in his life that he really wants to heal and make a big difference in their life. I gave him my number and told him to get into my web site.

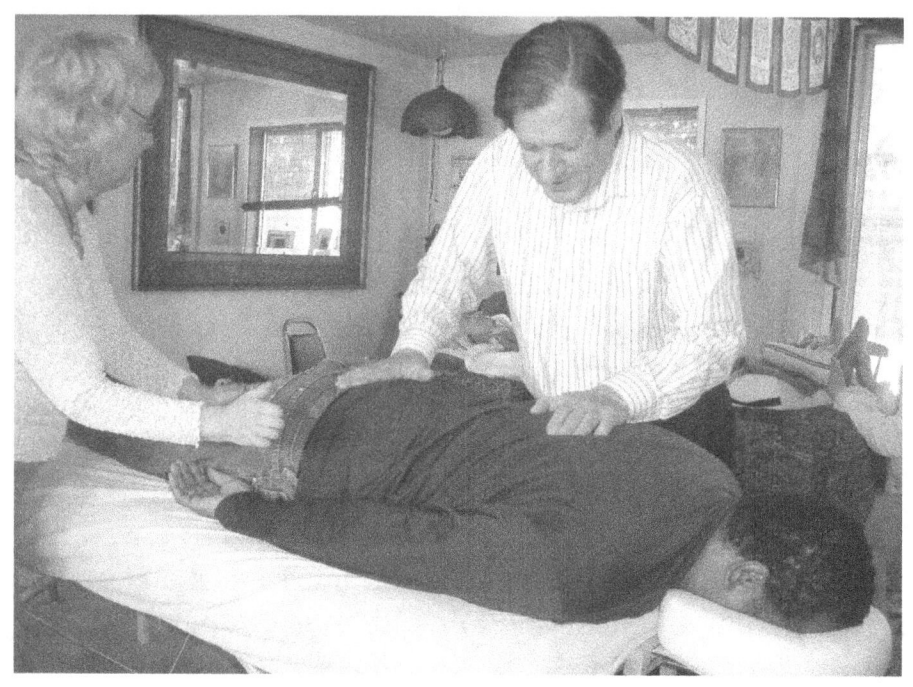

This photo is of our healing center in Willow Glen, part of San Jose, California. In the photo is Paul Barbaro, his wonderful, talented assistant Mona Angel, and a friend named Robert.

Bio of Author, Paul Barbaro

Paul Barbaro is an author of four books, speaker, health researcher, and longevity coach. He studied Psychology, languages, education and has a BS degree from UC Riverside, California.

Paul is an "Angel Whisperer." Paul channels your angels to help in your healing. He is an avid medical researcher. His strength is that he knows what he is looking for and does not quit until he finds it. Paul's persistence keeps him looking only for those things that work consistently well. Paul's healing system was given to him by two Native American (First Nation) Indian shamans. Paul had a thriving healing practice in 2008, and when he added this healing system to his practice, his healing results and client satisfaction went through the roof!

Throughout my journey I have come back to realize that true knowledge can only be uncovered from within myself; balanced by mind, body and spirit, driven by my hearts conscious expression for love towards all things.

Ultimately, my true purpose is to move into and with the true frequencies of our natural cosmic universe, using heart as my compass and engine. Still I continue to research, practice and transpose with such passion. Love is my work and my passion. Love is so close to Light that they seem to be the same. There is only one Light and one Truth (capital "T"). All Truth aligns with all other Truth. This makes your life much easier when seeking Truth. If it does not align with other Truths, it probably is not true."

Paul continues his research and healing work in Cupertino, California, and people interested in Paul's healing magic can call and make appointments. One does need to come to California, and stay for awhile. Healers that have a practice or spa can learn to do this healing system and boost their results and client satisfaction. There are training classes available in California. Paul presents informative, entertaining, enlightening, and captivating talks, lectures and presentations! Please call to book Mr. Barbaro for your next event.

Our Donation Hotline Phone Number:

1 (408) 253-6577

You can help to support us and our work. We can accept donations from all over the United States. We can use cars, SUV's, RV's, trucks, real estate, trusts, stock and trading accounts, boats, timeshares, jewelry, coin and stamp collections, antiques, and other things of value. We are applying for tax exempt status and we appreciate your support and donations. Please use this number for donations.

Thank you for buying and reading this book. It is important to get this information out into the real world.

It is okay with us for you to buy ten copies or more of this book and give them out to friends, family members, people in the healing arts and total strangers. For deep discounts on large orders, please call this office because we can sell the books lower than the list price. I hope this helps.

Thank You.

Sincerely,

Paul Barbaro, - Health Researcher, Pioneer and Author

OUTTAKES, Feb 21, 2016;

Notes on American and European Law

I believe and teach that the healing and restoration of our American land is linked to and re-establishing the languages, customs and societies of our Native peoples. The European mentality of slash, burn, scorch, cut, and plow under has reached the high achievement where we are now! In a mess, and things seem to be escalating for the worse especially in the Middle East. Remember these are out-takes. Not to be printed.

I am not an attorney, and this is not legal advice. I was once in business, and I was told, "Ignorance of the law is no excuse." So I figured I needed to study and know the law. When one wants legal advice one needs a licensed attorney to advise them. Again, this is not legal advice. In Forty years of study this is what I found. The years add prospective. **This is only for comedy-entertainment purposes.**

The entirety of American and European land law is that "He who gets there first owns the land and calls the shots." Look it up for yourself. This is what the race to the moon and to Mars is all about. Do you remember when Brittan was making a rush to the South Pole in the early 1900's? That is what it is all about. So the question is "How did the invading European's get around this law when they realized the value of Native American land.? They went out of their way to make sure everyone was taught that Native Americans, and Blacks, and the Chinese were not human! Can you imagine that? It was like taking away land from an animal, or plant! The issue now is that the law still is, "He who gets there first owns the land and calls the shots." So where does that put the Native Americans and all indigenous peoples? Please run all of this by an attorney who you trust before you do any of this. Please read on,

There are laws on the books that say when a treaty is violated, then there is no treaty at all. Now if one has ever seen the movie, "The Big Short" one sees that all of our financial and political regulatory systems are a "Free for All" as public policy. So then one asks the shocking and electrifying question, "Where did the Constitution and the law go?" because it is not here?" Good question! The good news is that, there is still an original law that is good. Just, there is no one doing it. And they call themselves the government, but there is a problem with that.

There are at least two US Constitutions, a real one and a fake one. Each state in the Union also has two Constitutions, a real one and a fake one! How did this happen? In the late 1800's upon one printing the ruling class simply re-printed the fake and they called it the real one, and no one noticed! A brilliant stroke of genius! But why would they do such a thing? And why aren't people more honest, and what's going on anyway? And what do they have to gain by fooling the people ruled by them. Well, you're in for a surprise! You get the mess that we are in right now! Lucky you!

Now how could we let it get that bad? Didn't the founding fathers tell you that if you slept on your rights you were going to loose them? Well that's what happened since 1864!

Here's How it Comes Down, If they ever drag you into their cesspool of a court room here it is;

All the valid legal arguments are a jurisdictional challenge. You must prepare your jurisdictional challenge from the first point of contact.
They can't hear the case because there is no proof before the private corporation court that you belong to, nor are subject to the private corporation codes, nor courts.

Yes! The courts all the way up to the U. S. Supreme Court are private corporation courts. And all the codes are private corporation codes. Their only job is to protect the corporation, the corporation codes, the fraud and the racketeering, because it makes them billions! Lucky them! You are not a part of the corporation. You have no standing in a corporation court, and they have no standing in a corporation court, plus they have no jurisdiction. A fake judge saying he has jurisdiction is not proof of jurisdiction. You want it in writing. If they give you a written document, you have proof of fraud and an action against them for damages.

The fake "government" rules by your consent. The moment you "consent" to their trap you can't win. They rule by your consent. I don't understand why people can't/don't understand that. In twenty years people will start using this argument, Why will they not research it now and use it now? To plead anything else is putting your head in the guillotine and cutting the rope holding the blade. I am starting to believe that "We the People" really enjoy spending years in the private corporation jail! Other wise why would you step into the court's rigged trap?

And you say you believe in "Liberty" when few even can grasp what that is. Challenge the court to produce the documents that prove that it has any constitutional foundation at all. Without those documents in the court room there is no jurisdiction. You want the proof in your hand, not the shabby word of the private corporation fake "judge." They can't and won't produce it in writing because they know that what they are doing is fraud. Those people who persist in the jurisdictional challenge win. Those that don't, loose. You keep pushing the jurisdictional challenge until you win. The "judge can not start a proceeding without establishing jurisdiction. Get into Google, or "findlaw.com" and research it.

I hope you realize that all the news reports are like Hollywood movie productions, esp. all the fears of ethnic groups, immigrants and terrorism. And the facts that the government has everything under control! It's starting to feel like they really want to start WWIII just like they started most of the other recent wars to make profits at the cost of young lives. Don't look now but wars cost many billions of dollars and someone is getting that money! Lucky them! And you and yours get the joy of going there to fight and die for the private corporation! Makes you proud, doesn't it? Your death for their billions, and for their agenda that they call "Freedom!" A wonderful deal for you! Ha!

I believe all the courts are corporations, and are owned by HSBC, in Shanghai, and London. It is hard to know who owns them. Try and find out for yourself. I hope not Afghanistan, Russia, Syria, China, nor Iran! Please if you can research this and let me know. That would really help.

When you demand to see the legal documents that prove the courts are constitutional, they can't do it because they are not. At that point jurisdiction has failed and you walk out of the court room. You have an absolute right to written proof that the court has jurisdiction, not just the say so of the dishonest/criminal "judge," who is a fake and he knows it. And you have an absolute right to a constitutional court from a legitimate constitutional government. And so far, that doesn't exist on Earth.

Impersonating a government officer is a felony! The fake "prosecutors" are the cream of the scum! They all know it is fake and a scam! And "the People" in who's name they prosecute you, is another fake private corporation. Please research this for your own state and let me know what you find. They get you by putting up a nice disguise or "smoke screen." And when you consent, they got you! We taxpayers pay the hundreds of billions of dollars a month to keep the scam going! Isn't our freedom wonderful! So precious that we put it in the toilet everyday, and laugh at it when we pull the handle to flush it, and then we wonder why things are so bad! I Love it! God Bless America. We all need it! And we feel we are "Safe." And that the politicos have it all under control!

A recent "government" scam is offering a free people a contract like a license or a "treaty." The trick is that license/treaty is a contract to perform to their whim. All court cases are for a failure to perform on a valid contract. Draw up a document that says you rescind your signature on all contracts, known of and unknown, for all time. And serve it on them so as to give them "Public Notice." This is not all the pieces of the trap/puzzle, I will let you know as the rest is discovered.

There is a subject called "Truth". Persistent use of the internet is used for finding the real truth. There is an art to finding the truth that you are looking for. It is now okay to seek the truth. Others are doing it, why not you?

Google and Youtube "Ces Qui Vie" trust and read and watch everything you can. It's a real eye opener. You are the EXECUTOR of this "Ces Qui Vie" trust. Pronounced "Sess Key Vie Trust." Your Liberty/freedom depends on this.

The correct statement is "I'm not challenging you, but jurisdiction is challenged and not proven in writing." "I have a right to written proof in my hand that you have jurisdiction." "Your saying that you have jurisdiction is not proof. I want proof." If the corporation "judge" proceeds without proof, you serve him with an affidavit of fraud and you ask the marshal to take him into custody as you will press felony fraud charges.

"To argue with a man who has renounced the use and authority of reason, and whose philosophy consists in holding humanity in contempt, is like administering medicine to the dead, or endeavoring to convert an atheist by scripture. Thomas Paine

www.ingramcontent.com/pod-product-compliance
Lightning Source LLC
Chambersburg PA
CBHW080412290526
45791CB00008BA/2243

* 9 7 8 1 4 9 5 3 7 3 6 0 2 *